The Visual Nurse's Basic Cardiac Rhythms Workbook

Tyler C. Scanlon, MS, BSN, RN

Registered Nurse, Cardiac Stress Lab

Guest Lecturer, Applied Exercise Physiology Department

University of Central Florida, Orlando, Florida

NOTICE

The criteria expressed in this book are based upon a consensus of previously published literature and texts in addition to the author's own experience and viewpoints. Readers are encouraged to seek additional references regarding ECG interpretation to continually improve their skills. The use of any devices or drugs should be preceded by careful review of their respective package inserts, which provide indications and dosages as approved by the USFDA. Readers are explicitly encouraged to consult package inserts prior to administration of any therapeutic agents. The author, editor, and publisher disclaim responsibility for adverse effects resulting from omissions and undetected errors or adverse results obtained from the use of the information in this book. Application of the information presented in a particular situation remains the professional responsibility of the licensed individual performing interventions. Information presented in this text is not medical advice and it is the responsibility of the reader to verify accuracy of all materials presented.

Thanks for picking up a copy!

If you're reading this, you're someone looking for a little more practice. Maybe you've already purchased a copy of The Visual Nurse's first publication, "Basic Cardiac Rhythms: The Visual Nurse's Guide" (and if so, thank you!). Or perhaps, you've used various other ECG & rhythm interpretation texts and found that there simply aren't enough sample strips to work through after the information is presented.

Unfortunately, many existing publications that teach cardiac rhythm interpretation fall short in the department of practice strips after presentation of the didactic material. This is no fault of the previous sources mentioned since this is not an easy task to accomplish.

That's where this workbook comes in. Because of the existing gap between information presentation and practical application related to rhythm interpretation, I received countless messages almost daily from students, new nurses and other medical professionals asking for a workbook that would help them actually APPLY what they've been taught.

The goal here is simple and straightforward

I'm going to assume that one of two things is true. 1) You've already got a foundational understanding of cardiac rhythms and are looking to master your interpretation skills from a *basic* rhythms perspective (this means that we're not covering topics like SVT with aberrant conductions versus VT, etc... you'd need a 12-lead ECG for that anyway) or 2) You're just beginning to learn about cardiac rhythms and dysrhythmias and are looking to apply what you learn as you go. In either case, this is the perfect workbook for you. Welcome, and I'm glad that you've trusted me to help you along the way. Thank you.

One note: A quick, down and dirty review of the cardiac cycle and normative values is presented in the following section but after that, we're going to jump right into what you came here for... THE RHYTHMS.

-Tyler, The Visual Nurse

Instagram & social: @thevisualnurse
YouTube.com/thevisualnurse
www.thevisualnurse.com

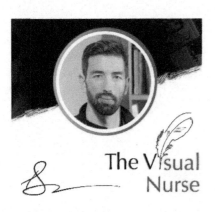

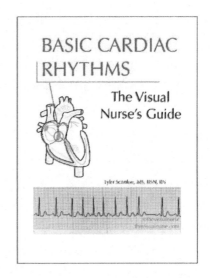

If you haven't already, check out the companion text available on Amazon (above)!

Table of Contents

THE CARDIAC CYCLE

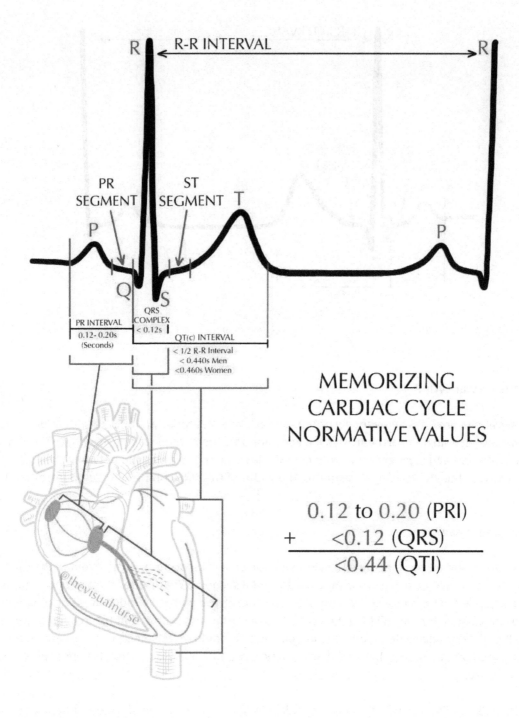

R-R INTERVAL

R

R

PR SEGMENT

ST SEGMENT

T

P

P

P

Q

S

QRS COMPLEX
< 0.12s

PR INTERVAL
0.12- 0.20s
(Seconds)

QT(c) INTERVAL

< 1/2 R-R Interval
< 0.440s Men
<0.460s Women

@thevisualnurse

MEMORIZING CARDIAC CYCLE NORMATIVE VALUES

$$
\begin{array}{r}
0.12 \text{ to } 0.20 \text{ (PRI)} \\
+ \quad <0.12 \text{ (QRS)} \\
\hline
<0.44 \text{ (QTI)}
\end{array}
$$

A SINGLE CARDIAC CYCLE

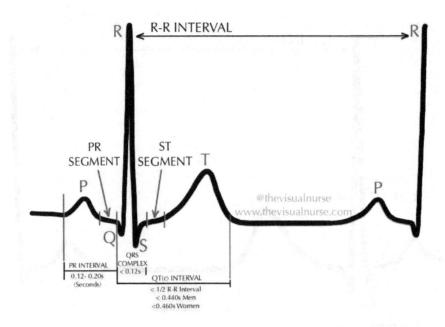

What is the cardiac cycle?

The graphic above provides an overview of the cardiac cycle, essentially a fancy term that describes the events composing a single heartbeat. This includes not only the named waveforms (PQRST) but also the associated intervals and segments that connect and describe the relationship between these wave forms. These are: the PR interval, PR segment, the width of the QRS complex, ST segment, and QT interval.

What does this mean?

Each wave and segment has a name and event with which it is associated. Every event in the cycle also has a normal range and each occurs within fractions of a second. What's important to understand is that each cardiac cycle *SHOULD* produce a pulse. For example, if you palpate a radial pulse on a patient you should feel a rebound for each QRS in the cycle. This describes the notion that mechanical (a pulse that can be felt indicating adequate blood flow and perfusion) should match electrical (the cardiac cycle or beat that's seen on the monitor). If a cardiac cycle occurs and a pulse is not felt, that beat likely did not perfuse adequately.

This is often easy to identify when taking a manual blood pressure as well. If a patient has frequent premature ventricular contractions you'll often hear a pause with each PVC on auscultation. This is because PVCs may or may not eject enough blood volume for adequate perfusion. This is the danger associated with sustained (>30 seconds) ventricular tachycardia.

Why should we care?

Each measurement and segment play an important role in cardiac rhythm interpretation. In order to recognize what is abnormal we have to know what the normal cycle looks like first, in textbook form. From these intervals, we can then build on this foundation and cover the most common (and some uncommon) telemetry rhythms that you'll come across. Rhythm interpretation is one of the most challenging topics for new nurses, paramedics, and medical residents, but it doesn't have to be! Next, let's take a look at each component of the cardiac cycle.

TAKE HOME POINTS

- ✓ The cardiac cycle represents a single heart beat
- ✓ Each cardiac cycle should produce a pulse
- ✓ If a cardiac cycle occurs and a pulse is not felt, that beat did not perfuse adequately

The P wave

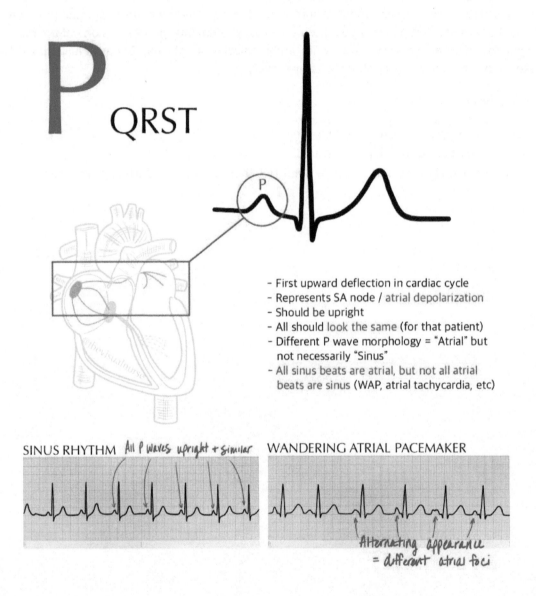

- First upward deflection in cardiac cycle
- Represents SA node / atrial depolarization
- Should be upright
- All should look the same (for that patient)
- Different P wave morphology = "Atrial" but not necessarily "Sinus"
- All sinus beats are atrial, but not all atrial beats are sinus (WAP, atrial tachycardia, etc)

SINUS RHYTHM   All P waves upright + similar

WANDERING ATRIAL PACEMAKER

Alternating appearance = different atrial foci

What is the P wave?

First to the party: the P wave. The P wave is the first positive deflection in the cardiac cycle (PQRST) and represents sino-atrial (SA) node and atrial (left *and* right sides) depolarization. This is important because the SA node is what we refer to as the natural "pacemaker" of the heart. It quite literally sets the pace for the timing of each cardiac cycle.

What does this mean?

All P waves should be upright and appear the same (for a specific patient anyway). My P waves may look different than yours, and yours may look different than your sister's. What's important is that your P waves all look the same and that they arrive 60 to 100 times per minute. If a P wave appears that looks different than the rest, we refer to it as an "atrial ectopic" beat. Ectopic simply means *from an abnormal origin*. The reason ectopic beats originating elsewhere in the atria appear differently from sinus P waves is because they take an alternate path to reach the atrio-ventricular (AV) node and ventricles. This alternate path means the electrode that's "watching" this electrical activity "sees" it differently.

If the impulse is traveling away from a positive electrode, the impulse will appear negative or *inverted*. If it's travelling perpendicular to the positive electrode then it may appear *biphasic*, meaning partially negative and partially positive. If an atrial beat comes early, we call it a premature atrial contraction (PAC). Premature atrial contractions are typically benign but may be felt as occasional palpitations in some patients.

What do we mean by sinus versus atrial? Think of it this way: all sinus beats are atrial but not all atrial beats are sinus. Why? Because the SA is located *within* the right atria. Case in point: the *wandering atrial pacemaker* rhythm strip shown below. No, this has nothing to with hardware or cardiac devices (i.e. implantable cardiac pacemakers). Instead, this rhythm refers to multiple atrial sites competing with one another to take the lead on setting the pace for the cardiac cycle. As a result, we see multiple P wave morphologies that appear different from one another.

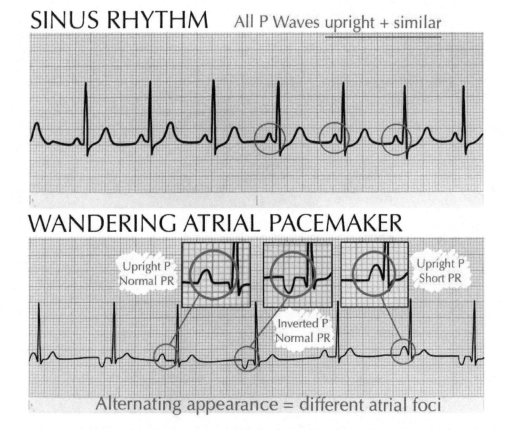

Why should we care?

In the case of the wandering atrial pacemaker the patient has multiple atrial foci that are depolarizing. Because of this, all P waves do not look the same. In this case we can't name the rhythm as sinus. Instead, we call it a wandering atrial pacemaker because the pacemaker of the heart is "wandering" throughout the atria (not really, but it describes the absence of a true set sinus pacemaker).

TAKE HOME POINTS

- ✓ The P wave is the first positive deflection in the cardiac cycle and represent atrial depolarization and contraction
- ✓ The SA node is referred to as the pacemaker of the heart
- ✓ All sinus beats are atrial but not all atrial beats are sinus

The P-R interval and PR segment

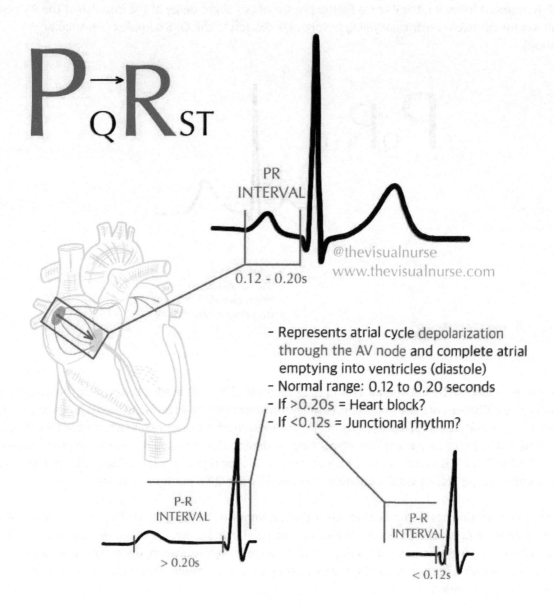

PR
INTERVAL

0.12 - 0.20s

@thevisualnurse
www.thevisualnurse.com

- Represents atrial cycle depolarization through the AV node and complete atrial emptying into ventricles (diastole)
- Normal range: 0.12 to 0.20 seconds
- If >0.20s = Heart block?
- If <0.12s = Junctional rhythm?

P-R
INTERVAL

> 0.20s

P-R
INTERVAL

< 0.12s

Following (and encompassing) the P wave is the P-R interval.

What is the P-R interval?

This part of the cardiac cycle describes the time needed for the impulse to leave the SA node and arrive/pass through the AV node. The PR interval represents the initiation of atrial depolarization (the P wave) and ends with depolarization through to the AV node (just before the QRS complex). It should be *constant* in length and between 0.12 and 0.20 seconds.

What does this mean?

During this time, the atria are fully contracting and emptying into the ventricles. In fact, the iso-electric (flat) P-R *segment* following the P wave (below) represents a slight delay of the impulse at the AV node. This allows for *complete ventricular filling* before progression to the QRS complex (ventricular activation).

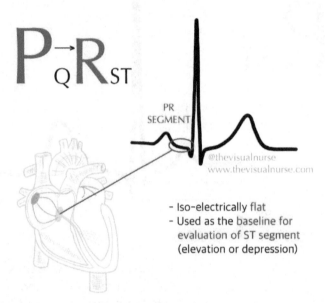

The P-R *interval* should be between 0.12 and 0.20 seconds. If it's less than 0.12 seconds the impulse is not likely sinus. Chances are the impulse is coming from somewhere in or near the AV junction (the area between the SA and AV node) since it's taking less time to reach the ventricles (where the QRS should begin). The P wave may be upright, inverted, or non-existent. But how could the P wave possibly be non-existent? If the P wave is inverted, it may be before the QRS or right after the QRS. If it's nowhere to be found it's likely to be *hidden* within and overshadowed by the QRS, but it's still there.

Rule #1 of interpreting basic cardiac rhythms is that an impulse traveling *toward a positive* electrode will produce a *positive (upward) deflection.* If your impulse is starting downstream (somewhere between the SA and AV node; in the junctional area) then it will have to travel *backward*, upstream to activate the part of the upper atria for which the SA node was originally responsible. This is called *retrograde* (backward) depolarization.

And if Rule #1 is that a *positive* impulse travelling toward a *positive* electrode produces a *positive* (upright) deflection, then a positive impulse travelling *away* from a positive electrode will produce a *negative* deflection. This is why *inverted* P waves with a short PR interval are said to be junctional; they originate from the AV junction, or area between the SA and the AV node and travel backward while the rest of the impulse heads toward the ventricles as it usually would. Think of it as sending a messenger to the upper atria while you continue to head toward the ventricles.

If the P-R interval is greater than 0.20 seconds, it's likely that you're looking at an atrio-ventricular block (AVB), meaning that for some reason the impulse is taking its sweet time to reach the ventricles. The P-R interval may be long and constant (1st degree AV block), variable and lengthening with each beat (2nd degree type 1), or in total disconnect and unrelated to the QRS (complete / 3rd degree AVB).

Why should we care?

The P-R interval provides clues as to where supraventricular beats are originating and what the relationship is between those beats and the ventricles below. This can all be inferred based upon the time relationship between the two. Next up let's take a look at the QRS complex and ventricular activation.

TAKE HOME POINTS

- ✓ The PR interval describes the time needed for the impulse to leave the SA node and arrive/ pass through the AV node
- ✓ The PR interval should be *constant* in length and between 0.12 and 0.20 seconds.
- ✓ Less than 0.12 seconds may indicate a junctional origin
- ✓ Greater than 0.20 seconds may indicate an AV block or impulse delay
- ✓ Inverted P waves indicate retrograde (backward) atrial depolarization

The QRS complex

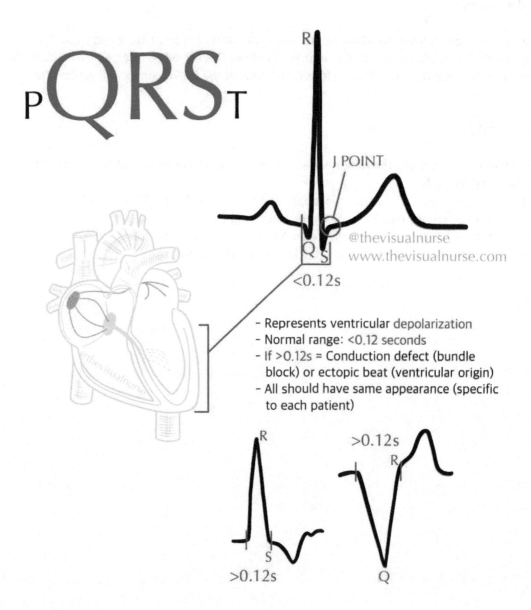

P**QRS**T

R

J POINT

@thevisualnurse
www.thevisualnurse.com

Q S
<0.12s

- Represents ventricular depolarization
- Normal range: <0.12 seconds
- If >0.12s = Conduction defect (bundle block) or ectopic beat (ventricular origin)
- All should have same appearance (specific to each patient)

R

S
>0.12s

>0.12s

R

Q

The QRS complex. We've made it to the ventricles.

What is the QRS complex?

Following a slight delay at the AV node the electrical impulse is ready to travel down the bundle of His, into to the left and right bundle branches, and terminally to the purkinje fibers. The QRS complex represents this, indicating depolarization and contraction of the ventricles.

What does this mean?

This complex is short in duration (≤ 0.12 seconds). This is largely thanks to the purkinje fibers through which the impulse travels tremendously fast. This is important. The ventricles are relatively thick and need to depolarize simultaneously throughout to allow as much blood as possible to be expelled.

In cases where the QRS complex is greater than 0.12 seconds, the ventricles are taking longer to depolarize which is inefficient. If it's a single, early, wide beat on the ECG, it may be a premature ventricular contraction (PVC). If they come as 3-4 or more successively, you may be looking at ventricular tachycardia, a potentially lethal rhythm if sustained (aberrant bundle branch block conduction may also cause this but is beyond the current scope). With sustained inefficient beats at a high rate, ejection fraction decreases, filling time is impaired, cardiac output is decreased, and blood supply to the heart decreases via the coronary arteries during diastole.

Why should I care?

Rapid rates with a wide cardiac conduction time also increases the oxygen demand on the heart potentially leading to ischemia, progressing myocardial injury, and patient deterioration. Understanding why a narrow QRS is important as well as the ability to recognize a wide QRS will help in appreciating the importance of frequent wide and bizarre looking complexes when analyzing rhythm strips in the future.

TAKE HOME POINTS

- ✓ The QRS complex represents ventricular depolarization and contraction
- ✓ The QRS should measure ≤ 0.12 seconds
- ✓ Wide QRS complexes are relatively inefficient contractions
- ✓ Wide QRS beats at a very rapid rate may be lethal, if sustained and negatively affecting hemodynamic stability

The J point and ST segment

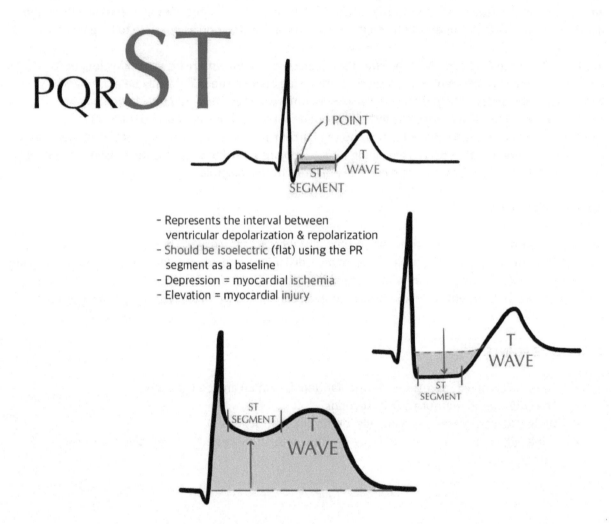

- Represents the interval between ventricular depolarization & repolarization
- Should be isoelectric (flat) using the PR segment as a baseline
- Depression = myocardial ischemia
- Elevation = myocardial injury

What is the ST segment?

Following the QRS complex is the ST segment. Before looking at this diagnostic segment we should first understand the *J point*. The J point is the point at which the S wave of the QRS makes the turn to head back to baseline (J joins the S with the T). This is important because this marks the beginning of the ST segment.

The normal ST segment should be flat (isoelectric) at baseline. We evaluate this by using the PR segment (or sometimes the P-Q junction with rapid heart rates) as the isoelectric starting point. Remember that the PR *segment* represents the point at which the atria have fully contracted and the heart is now electrically *neutral*. To evaluate if the ST segment falls above, in line, or below the PR segment draw a straight, horizontal line from one to the other. Generally speaking, one small box (0.04 seconds; 1 mm) above or below the isoelectric line is considered abnormal.

What does this mean?

ST segment depression may represent myocardial ischemia (impaired oxygen delivery). ST segment elevation may warn of potential tissue injury and tissue death if untreated (the famed *STEMI*; ST elevation myocardial infarction). Broadly speaking, the injury is likely to kill you first (elevation), but both should be treated with the same respect since each may rapidly progress to deterioration. Of course, certain chronic conditions may cause ST segment depression (such as left ventricular strain pattern) and elevation (benign early repolarization, pericarditis, Brugada syndrome, etc.). Regardless, grab a prior ECG for comparison if available and always treat the patient, not the monitor. The monitor is simply there to provide context to the overall clinical picture.

ST segment elevation and depression are described partly in terms of millimeters. The smallest box on the ECG paper is 0.04 seconds in duration, and 1mm in length and height.

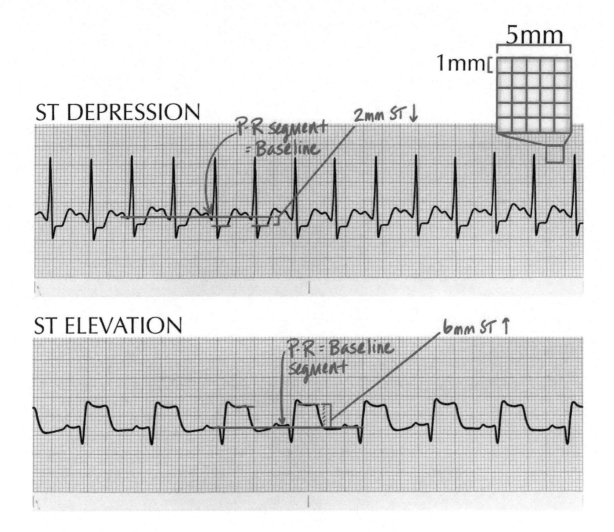

Why should we care?

The ST segment is one of the strongest diagnostic considerations when a patient is experiencing chest pain or other veiled symptoms. Women and diabetics in particular may not always report chest pain as anginal equivalents. Nausea, jaw pain, and other symptoms may be ominous presentations that should be clinically correlated with ECG findings. Symptomatic ST changes must be treated accordingly and the pain must resolve completely. The key is to compare to a previous ECG when possible and to collect serial ECGs which may show trends over time.

TAKE HOME POINTS

- ✓ The J point is the point at which the S wave of the QRS makes the turn to head back to baseline and marks the beginning of the ST segment
- ✓ The normal ST segment should be flat (isoelectric) and in line with the PR segment
- ✓ One small box above or below the PR segment should be considered abnormal
- ✓ ST segment depression indicates myocardial ischemia
- ✓ ST segment elevation indicates myocardial injury

The T wave

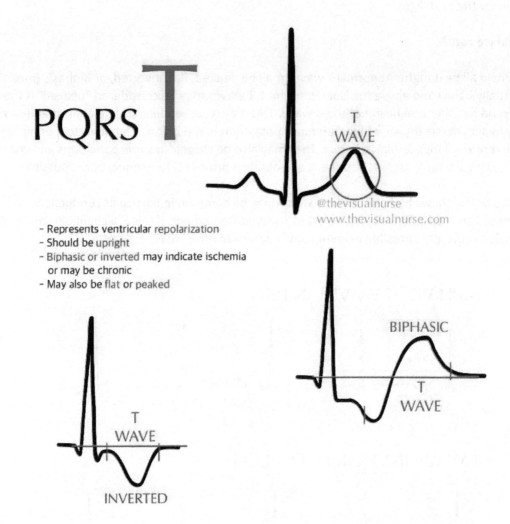

PQRS **T**

T WAVE

@thevisualnurse
www.thevisualnurse.com

- Represents ventricular repolarization
- Should be upright
- Biphasic or inverted may indicate ischemia
  or may be chronic
- May also be flat or peaked

BIPHASIC
T WAVE

T WAVE
INVERTED

What is the T wave?

The T wave represents ventricular relaxation and repolarization.

What does this mean?

At this point, the ventricles are refractory, meaning they're unable to respond to any incoming impulses and are not able to depolarize. During this period, the cells of the heart are in the process of recharging for the next impulse and wave of contraction. Sometimes, you may see a premature atrial beat (P wave) delivered and the ventricles will not respond. It can sometimes mimic a transient heart block so take a closer look. Essentially the ventricles are saying, "Nope, we just contracted and we're on break, so send another sinus beat in a few seconds and we'll pick that one up."

Refractory states are similar to the windshield wipers on your car. When the wipers are in the down-swing process of wiping, if you decide to bump the wiper signal to clear the windshield one more time, do the wipers stop half way and automatically go back up? No. They travel all the way back to resting before completing the next sweep that you signaled. This is the concept of refractoriness and this is the significance of the T wave; signifying the repolarization of the ventricles to their resting state in preparation for the next signal.

Why should we care?

T waves should all be upright. Abnormal T waves may be peaked, flat, inverted, or biphasic (meaning they're partially below and above the isoelectric line). T waves may be considered "peaked" if they extend beyond half the total height of the R wave. This may represent electrolyte abnormalities, most commonly hyperkalemia (hyper = high, kalemia = potassium in the blood). Flat, inverted, or biphasic T waves may represent myocardial ischemia. They may also be chronic in some conditions and conduction abnormalities. In any case, assess the patient and obtain a prior ECG for comparison if possible.

The first ECG below shows biphasic T waves which may be common in particular conduction abnormalities. The second ECG depicts inverted T waves. Remember, if this is a change from baseline, T wave inversion represents possible ischemia until confirmed otherwise.

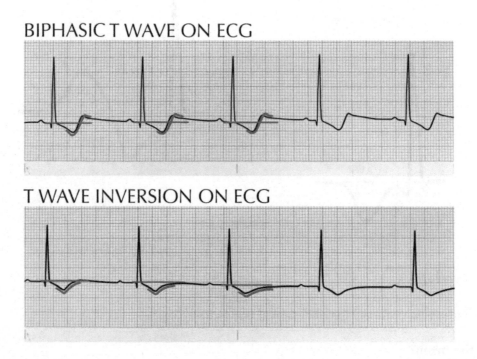

BIPHASIC T WAVE ON ECG

T WAVE INVERSION ON ECG

TAKE HOME POINTS:

- ✓ The T wave represents ventricular relaxation and repolarization
- ✓ Abnormal T waves may be peaked, flat, inverted, or biphasic
- ✓ Flat or inverted T waves may represent myocardial ischemia; assess the patient and correlate with the clinical picture

The QT interval

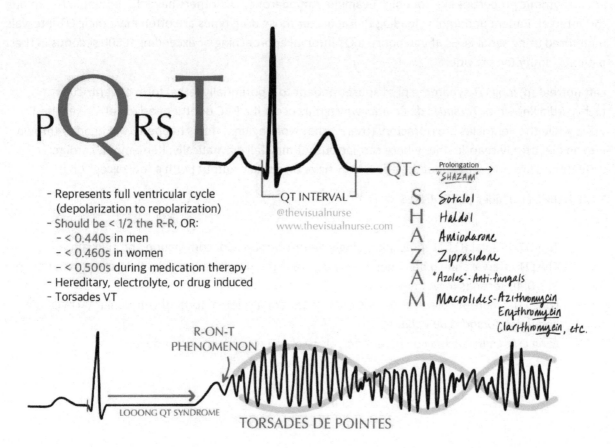

- Represents full ventricular cycle (depolarization to repolarization)
- Should be < 1/2 the R-R, OR:
  - < 0.440s in men
  - < 0.460s in women
  - < 0.500s during medication therapy
- Hereditary, electrolyte, or drug induced
- Torsades VT

QT INTERVAL
@thevisualnurse
www.thevisualnurse.com

QTc ——Prolongation——→ "SHAZAM"
S Sotalol
H Haldol
A Amiodarone
Z Ziprasidone
A "Azoles" - Anti-fungals
M Macrolides - Azithromycin
   Erythromycin
   Clarithromycin, etc.

R-ON-T PHENOMENON

LOOONG QT SYNDROME

TORSADES DE POINTES

What is the QT interval?

The QT interval (QTI) represents a single *ventricular* cycle of contraction and relaxation.

What does this mean?

If you recall the previous letters of the cardiac cycle and what each represents, this will tell you exactly what the QT interval is describing. The "Q" of the QRS complex represents the beginning of ventricular activation and contraction. The T wave represents ventricular relaxation and repolarization. Together, the QTI describes the time the entire process takes.

Speaking of time, what are the acceptable intervals for this measure? Broadly, the QT interval should be less than half the R to R interval. More specifically, the QTI should be ≤ 0.44 seconds in men, and ≤ 0.46 seconds in women. Women are known to have longer QT intervals when corrected for rate compared to their male counterparts, although the mechanism is not fully understood. Fortunately, it's not an *absolute* predictor for cardiac arrhythmias and sudden death. Wait, sudden death? Why are we talking about this?

Why should we care?

Long QT syndrome may be hereditary, electrolyte induced, or drug induced. In fact, medications with antiarrhythmic properties like Sotalol, Flecainide, Amiodarone, and others have the potential to prolong this interval. Patient undergoing loading therapies for these drug types are often have their QT intervals monitored using serial ECGs. If you notice a QT interval approaching or exceeding 0.500 seconds in these patients, notify the provider.

Left untreated, long QT syndrome predisposes patient to a potentially lethal form of ventricular tachycardia known as *Torsades de Pointes* which may occur if a PVC or other early beat strikes the T wave while the ventricles are refractory (there's that word again..) If this happens, the heart is thrown into an electrically chaotic state where cardiac output may fall dramatically. Remember, cardiac arrhythmias are primarily about the effect they have on cardiac output (with a few exceptions).

TAKE HOME (Torsades de) **POINTES:**

- ✓ The QT interval (QTI) represents a single *ventricular* cycle of contraction and relaxation
- ✓ The QT interval should be either 1) less than half the R to R interval 2) ≤ 0.44 seconds in men or 3) ≤ 0.46 seconds in women
- ✓ Long QT syndrome predisposes patient to a potentially lethal form of ventricular tachycardia known as *Torsades de Pointes*
- ✓ Long QT syndrome may be hereditary, electrolyte induced, or drug induced

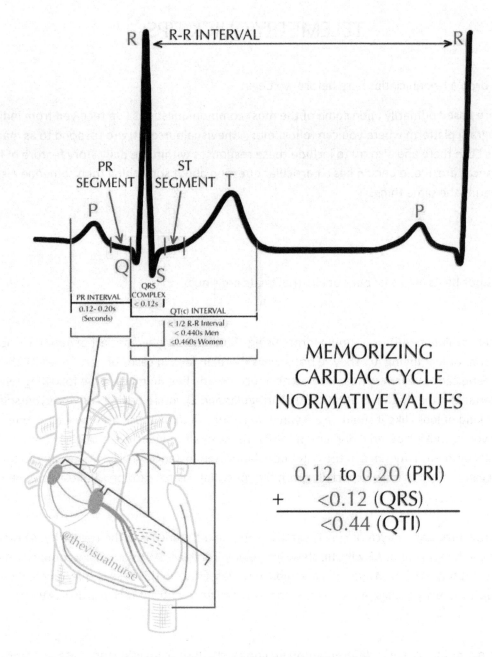

R-R INTERVAL

PR SEGMENT

ST SEGMENT

P

Q S

QRS COMPLEX < 0.12s

PR INTERVAL

0.12- 0.20s (Seconds)

QT(c) INTERVAL

< 1/2 R-R Interval
< 0.440s Men
<0.460s Women

T

P

R

R

@thevisualnurse

MEMORIZING
CARDIAC CYCLE
NORMATIVE VALUES

$$
\begin{array}{r}
0.12 \text{ to } 0.20 \ (\text{PRI}) \\
+ \quad <0.12 \ (\text{QRS}) \\
\hline
<0.44 \ (\text{QTI})
\end{array}
$$

This is the same image we saw at the beginning of the chapter. Hopefully we were able to tie each concept together sufficiently enough that you now see the story that the cardiac cycle tells. In the next section the practice strips are presented, followed by the answer key in the final section of the workbook.

TAKE HOME POINTS:

✓ Easily remember the norms for cardiac cycle intervals: 12 to 20 (PRI), less than 12 (QRS), add all three to get less than 44 (QT).

TELEMETRY QUICK TIPS

I wanted to drop a few quick tips here before we begin.

These tips are based primarily upon some of the most common questions I've received from individuals on the Instagram platform where you can follow me: @thevisualnurse. I try to respond to as many messages as I can there and also try to include these responses within the daily story feature of the page because chances are, if one person has a particular question about something then someone else is likely wondering the same thing.

Tip #1:

    ✓ All sinus beats are atrial but not all atrial beats are sinus.

Tip #2:

    ✓ Atrial fibrillation (AF): you should forget using "fibrillation waves" as part of your inclusion criteria for identifying AF. They're not always there. In fact, in cases of very "fine" AF the baseline can appear very near isoelectric. I recommend beginning with the following two criteria: 1) If the rhythm is IRREGULARLY irregular and 2) you're having convince yourself "well, that kind of looks like it could be a P wave there" or... "I *think* those are P waves..." then chances are you're looking at atrial fibrillation (other differentials may include WAP, MAT, etc.). It's the most common arrhythmia in the adult population and instances increase with age so this is one you can't afford to miss, especially given the potential risk for cardioembolic events, like stroke.

Tip #3:

    ✓ Supraventricular tachycardia (SVT) versus A-fib: the difference is in the regularity. At rapid rates this can be tough, but AF will still show irregularly irregular. SVT is a narrow complex regular rhythm above 150 BPM and no discernible P waves. (*SVT in this case is referring to AV-nodal re-entrant tachycardias (AVNRT) and atrio-ventricular re-entrant tachycardias (AVRT)).

Tip #4:

    ✓ The major difference in differentiation junctional rhythms from idioventricular rhythms is the width of the QRS. Narrow = junctional. Wide = ventricular.

Tip #5:

    ✓ Inverted P waves: If the P wave is inverted and the PR interval is normal, its atrial but not sinus (atrial ectopic). If the P wave is inverted and PR interval is short (<0.12s), its junctional.

Tip #6:

    ✓ All Torsades de Pointes (TdP) are a form of polymorphic VT but not all polymorphic VT qualify as Torsades. Remember that for TdP you must have evidence of a prolonged QT interval to make this call.

Tip #7:

✓ Complete heart blocks (CHB): the QRS isn't always wide. If the AV junction picks up the escape mechanism, the QRS will be narrow. If the junction fails and the ventricles initiate the escape, the QRS will be wide. Pay attention to the PR interval.

Tip #8:

✓ Heart rate (HR) calculations: for irregular rhythms I recommend using the 6 second method for calculating HR. Of course you could count the amount of small boxes between the two closest R waves and the two widest to find a HR range but why torture yourself with that? For extremely fast rhythms, consider using the big box method in the real world when an approximation is all that's needed and your patient needs treatment.

Tip #9:

✓ QTc: The QT interval is influenced by heart rates. Faster heart rates are associated with shortening QT intervals and slower heart rate are associated with lengthening QT intervals. In these cases it may be appropriate to describe the QT interval *corrected* for heart rate QT(c) (QT relative to what it *would measure* if the heart rate were 60 beats per minute). ECG machines routinely perform this measure automatically but for your own knowledge, the Bazett's formula is the most commonly recognized: QT/(the square root of the R-R interval).

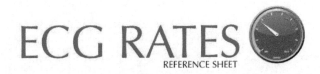

ECG RATES
REFERENCE SHEET

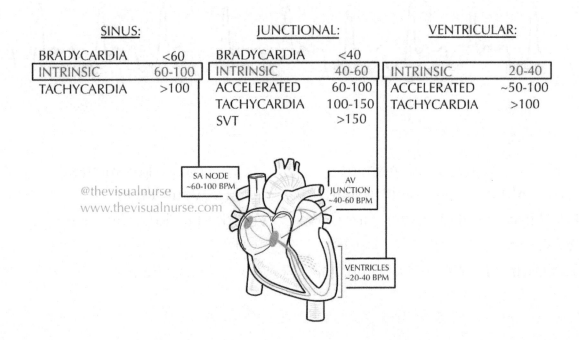

SINUS:		JUNCTIONAL:		VENTRICULAR:	
BRADYCARDIA	<60	BRADYCARDIA	<40		
INTRINSIC	60-100	INTRINSIC	40-60	INTRINSIC	20-40
TACHYCARDIA	>100	ACCELERATED	60-100	ACCELERATED	~50-100
		TACHYCARDIA	100-150	TACHYCARDIA	>100
		SVT	>150		

SA NODE
~60-100 BPM

AV JUNCTION
~40-60 BPM

VENTRICLES
~20-40 BPM

@thevisualnurse
www.thevisualnurse.com

PRACTICE STRIPS

1.

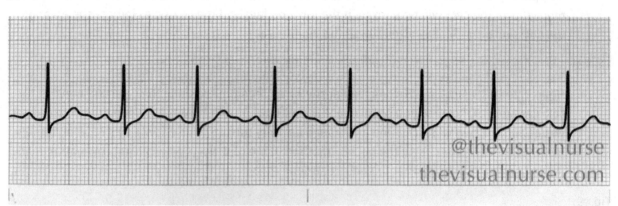

        (6 second method)   (Small box method)
RATE: Atrial: _____   Ventricular: _____   Ventricular: _____
RHYTHM: <u>Atrial</u> Regular Irregular   <u>Ventricular</u> Regular Irregular
P WAVES: _____   PR: _____   QRS: _____   QT: _____
ST SEGMENT: Okay Elevated Depressed   T WAVES: _____

2.

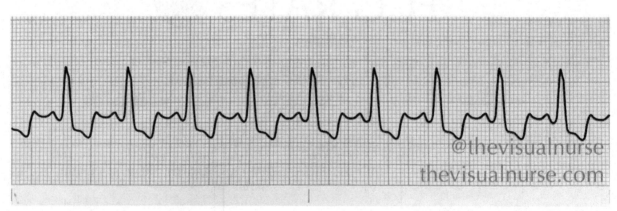

        (6 second method)   (Small box method)
RATE: Atrial: _____   Ventricular: _____   Ventricular: _____
RHYTHM: <u>Atrial</u> Regular Irregular   <u>Ventricular</u> Regular Irregular
P WAVES: _____   PR: _____   QRS: _____   QT: _____
ST SEGMENT: Okay Elevated Depressed   T WAVES: _____

3.

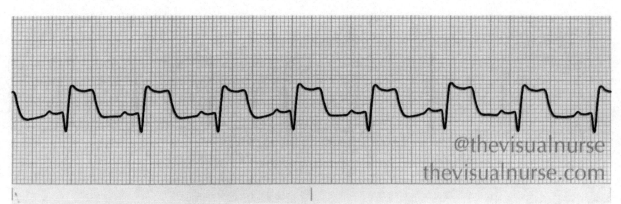

(6 second method)   (Small box method)

RATE: Atrial: _____   Ventricular: _____   Ventricular: _____

RHYTHM: <u>Atrial</u> Regular Irregular   <u>Ventricular</u> Regular Irregular

P WAVES: _____   PR: _____   QRS: _____   QT: _____

ST SEGMENT: Okay Elevated Depressed   T WAVES: _____

4.

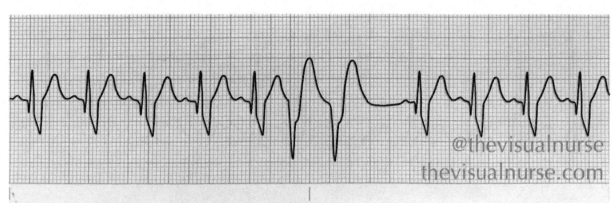

(6 second method)   (Small box method)

RATE: Atrial: _____   Ventricular: _____   Ventricular: _____

RHYTHM: <u>Atrial</u> Regular Irregular   <u>Ventricular</u> Regular Irregular

P WAVES: _____   PR: _____   QRS: _____   QT: _____

ST SEGMENT: Okay Elevated Depressed   T WAVES: _____

5.

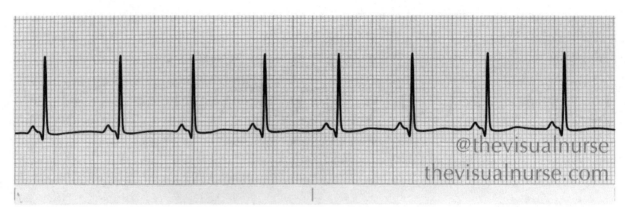

(6 second method)   (Small box method)

RATE: Atrial: _____   Ventricular: _____   Ventricular: _____

RHYTHM: <u>Atrial</u> Regular Irregular   <u>Ventricular</u> Regular Irregular

P WAVES: _____   PR: _____   QRS: _____   QT: _____

ST SEGMENT: Okay Elevated Depressed   T WAVES: _____

6.

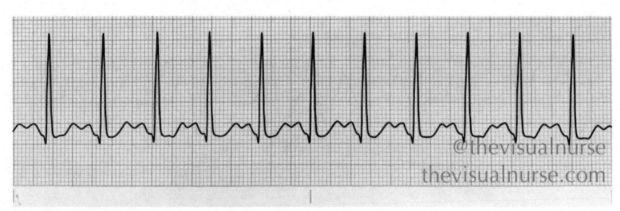

(6 second method)   (Small box method)

RATE: Atrial: _____   Ventricular: _____   Ventricular: _____

RHYTHM: <u>Atrial</u> Regular Irregular   <u>Ventricular</u> Regular Irregular

P WAVES: _____   PR: _____   QRS: _____   QT: _____

ST SEGMENT: Okay Elevated Depressed   T WAVES: _____

7.

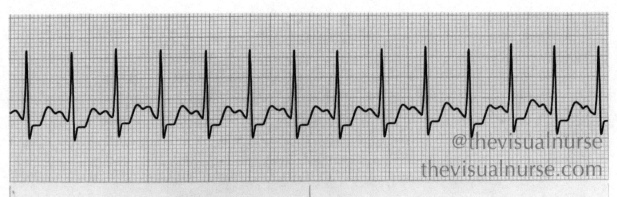

(6 second method)   (Small box method)
RATE: Atrial: _____   Ventricular: _____   Ventricular: _____
RHYTHM: Atrial Regular Irregular   Ventricular Regular Irregular
P WAVES: _____   PR: _____   QRS: _____   QT: _____
ST SEGMENT: Okay Elevated Depressed   T WAVES: _____

8.

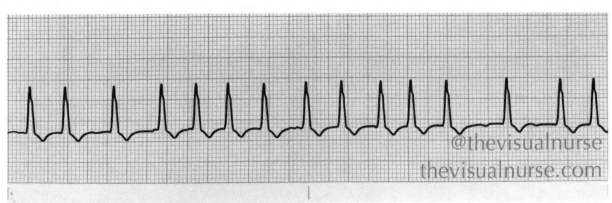

(6 second method)   (Small box method)
RATE: Atrial: _____   Ventricular: _____   Ventricular: _____
RHYTHM: Atrial Regular Irregular   Ventricular Regular Irregular
P WAVES: _____   PR: _____   QRS: _____   QT: _____
ST SEGMENT: Okay Elevated Depressed   T WAVES: _____

9.

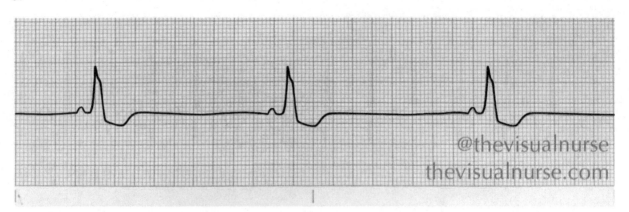

(6 second method)   (Small box method)

RATE: Atrial: _____ Ventricular: _____   Ventricular: _____

RHYTHM: <u>Atrial</u> Regular Irregular   <u>Ventricular</u> Regular Irregular

P WAVES: _____ PR: _____ QRS: _____ QT: _____

ST SEGMENT: Okay Elevated Depressed   T WAVES: _____

10.

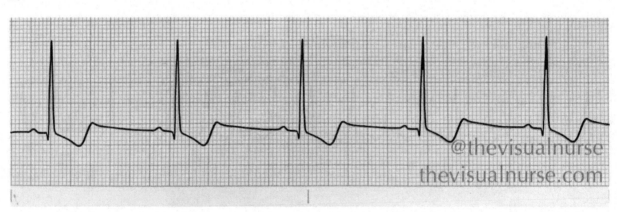

(6 second method)   (Small box method)

RATE: Atrial: _____ Ventricular: _____   Ventricular: _____

RHYTHM: <u>Atrial</u> Regular Irregular   <u>Ventricular</u> Regular Irregular

P WAVES: _____ PR: _____ QRS: _____ QT: _____

ST SEGMENT: Okay Elevated Depressed   T WAVES: _____

11.

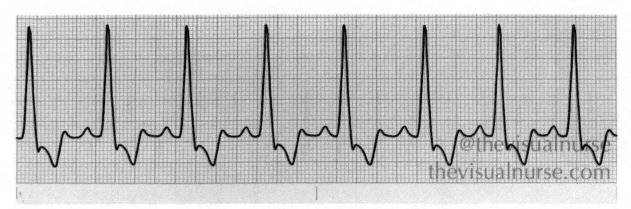

          (6 second method)   (Small box method)

RATE: Atrial: _____ Ventricular: _____   Ventricular: _____

RHYTHM: <u>Atrial</u> Regular Irregular   <u>Ventricular</u> Regular Irregular

P WAVES: _____ PR: _____ QRS: _____ QT: _____

ST SEGMENT: Okay Elevated Depressed   T WAVES: _____

12.

Patient resting comfortably, takes a deep breath then exhales

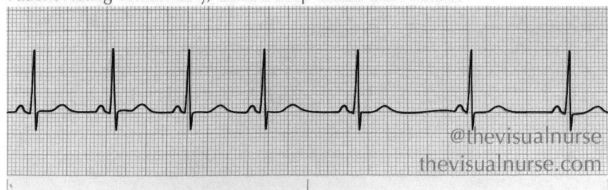

          (6 second method)   (Small box method)

RATE: Atrial: _____ Ventricular: _____   Ventricular: _____

RHYTHM: <u>Atrial</u> Regular Irregular   <u>Ventricular</u> Regular Irregular

P WAVES: _____ PR: _____ QRS: _____ QT: _____

ST SEGMENT: Okay Elevated Depressed   T WAVES: _____

13.

Patient resting comfortably. HR jumps rapidly & tracing below is present

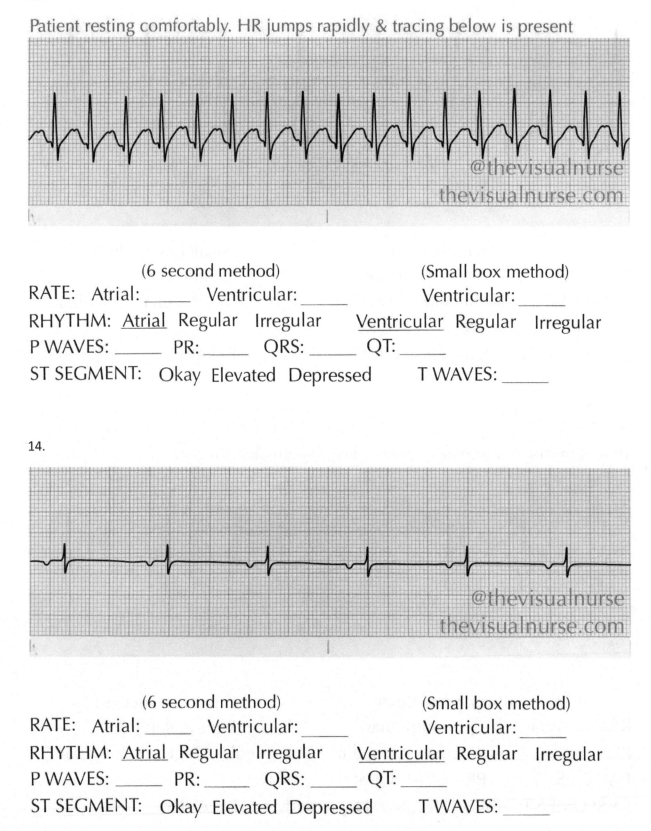

(6 second method)   (Small box method)
RATE: Atrial: _____   Ventricular: _____   Ventricular: _____
RHYTHM: <u>Atrial</u> Regular Irregular   <u>Ventricular</u> Regular Irregular
P WAVES: _____   PR: _____   QRS: _____   QT: _____
ST SEGMENT: Okay Elevated Depressed   T WAVES: _____

14.

(6 second method)   (Small box method)
RATE: Atrial: _____   Ventricular: _____   Ventricular: _____
RHYTHM: <u>Atrial</u> Regular Irregular   <u>Ventricular</u> Regular Irregular
P WAVES: _____   PR: _____   QRS: _____   QT: _____
ST SEGMENT: Okay Elevated Depressed   T WAVES: _____

15.

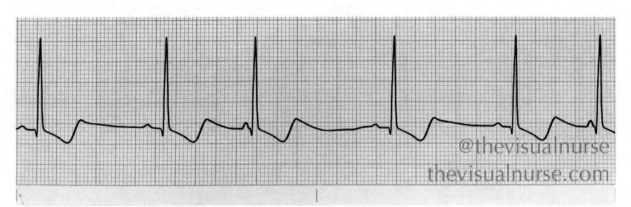

                 (6 second method)   (Small box method)
RATE: Atrial: _____   Ventricular: _____   Ventricular: _____
RHYTHM: <u>Atrial</u> Regular Irregular   <u>Ventricular</u> Regular Irregular
P WAVES: _____   PR: _____   QRS: _____   QT: _____
ST SEGMENT: Okay Elevated Depressed   T WAVES: _____

16.

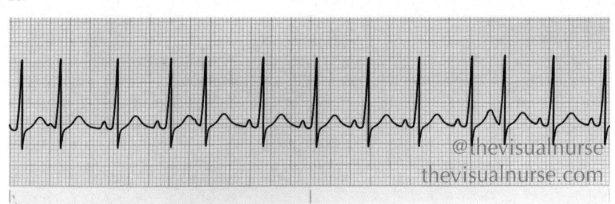

                 (6 second method)   (Small box method)
RATE: Atrial: _____   Ventricular: _____   Ventricular: _____
RHYTHM: <u>Atrial</u> Regular Irregular   <u>Ventricular</u> Regular Irregular
P WAVES: _____   PR: _____   QRS: _____   QT: _____
ST SEGMENT: Okay Elevated Depressed   T WAVES: _____

17.

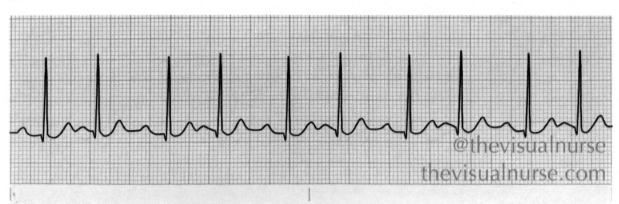

          (6 second method)   (Small box method)

RATE: Atrial: _____ Ventricular: _____   Ventricular: _____

RHYTHM: <u>Atrial</u> Regular Irregular   <u>Ventricular</u> Regular Irregular

P WAVES: _____ PR: _____ QRS: _____ QT: _____

ST SEGMENT: Okay Elevated Depressed   T WAVES: _____

18.

Patient resting comfortably, takes a deep breath and exhales slowly

          (6 second method)   (Small box method)

RATE: Atrial: _____ Ventricular: _____   Ventricular: _____

RHYTHM: <u>Atrial</u> Regular Irregular   <u>Ventricular</u> Regular Irregular

P WAVES: _____ PR: _____ QRS: _____ QT: _____

ST SEGMENT: Okay Elevated Depressed   T WAVES: _____

19.

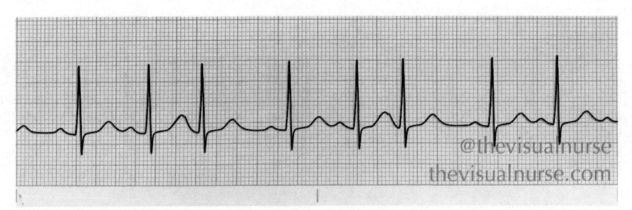

(6 second method)   (Small box method)

RATE: Atrial: _____   Ventricular: _____   Ventricular: _____

RHYTHM: <u>Atrial</u> Regular Irregular   <u>Ventricular</u> Regular Irregular

P WAVES: _____   PR: _____   QRS: _____   QT: _____

ST SEGMENT: Okay Elevated Depressed   T WAVES: _____

20.

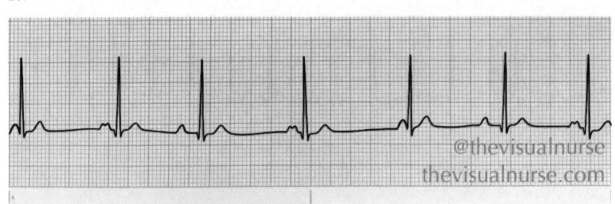

(6 second method)   (Small box method)

RATE: Atrial: _____   Ventricular: _____   Ventricular: _____

RHYTHM: <u>Atrial</u> Regular Irregular   <u>Ventricular</u> Regular Irregular

P WAVES: _____   PR: _____   QRS: _____   QT: _____

ST SEGMENT: Okay Elevated Depressed   T WAVES: _____

21.

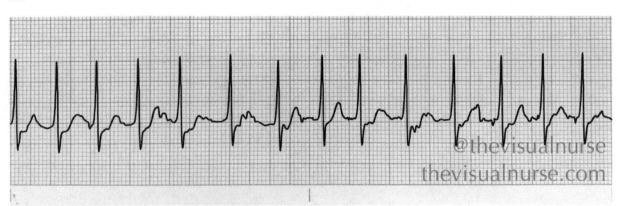

(6 second method)   (Small box method)

RATE: Atrial: _____   Ventricular: _____   Ventricular: _____

RHYTHM: <u>Atrial</u> Regular Irregular   <u>Ventricular</u> Regular Irregular

P WAVES: _____   PR: _____   QRS: _____   QT: _____

ST SEGMENT: Okay Elevated Depressed   T WAVES: _____

22.

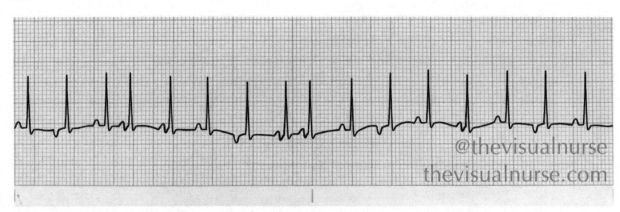

(6 second method)   (Small box method)

RATE: Atrial: _____   Ventricular: _____   Ventricular: _____

RHYTHM: <u>Atrial</u> Regular Irregular   Ventricular Regular Irregular

P WAVES: _____   PR: _____   QRS: _____   QT: _____

ST SEGMENT: Okay Elevated Depressed   T WAVES: _____

23.

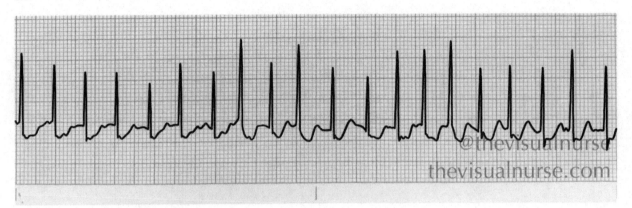

                    (6 second method)   (Small box method)
RATE: Atrial: _____   Ventricular: _____   Ventricular: _____
RHYTHM: <u>Atrial</u> Regular Irregular   <u>Ventricular</u> Regular Irregular
P WAVES: _____ PR: _____   QRS: _____   QT: _____
ST SEGMENT: Okay Elevated Depressed   T WAVES: _____

24.

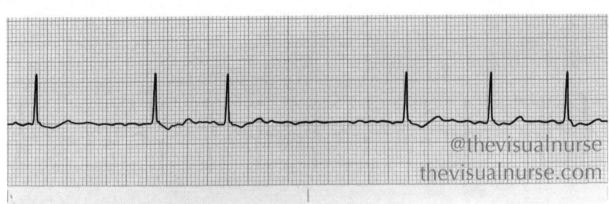

                    (6 second method)   (Small box method)
RATE: Atrial: _____   Ventricular: _____   Ventricular: _____
RHYTHM: <u>Atrial</u> Regular Irregular   <u>Ventricular</u> Regular Irregular
P WAVES: _____ PR: _____   QRS: _____   QT: _____
ST SEGMENT: Okay Elevated Depressed   T WAVES: _____

25.

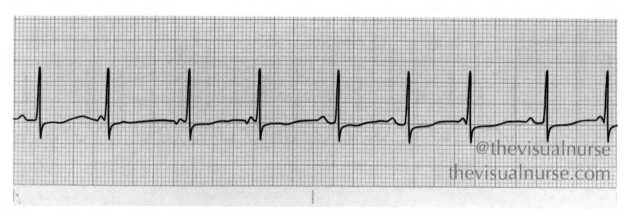

(6 second method)   (Small box method)

RATE: Atrial: _____   Ventricular: _____   Ventricular: _____

RHYTHM: <u>Atrial</u> Regular Irregular   <u>Ventricular</u> Regular Irregular

P WAVES: _____ PR: _____   QRS: _____   QT: _____

ST SEGMENT: Okay Elevated Depressed   T WAVES: _____

26.

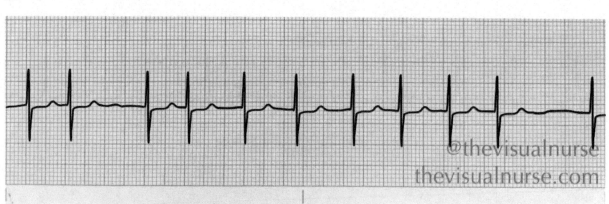

(6 second method)   (Small box method)

RATE: Atrial: _____   Ventricular: _____   Ventricular: _____

RHYTHM: <u>Atrial</u> Regular Irregular   <u>Ventricular</u> Regular Irregular

P WAVES: _____ PR: _____   QRS: _____   QT: _____

ST SEGMENT: Okay Elevated Depressed   T WAVES: _____

27.

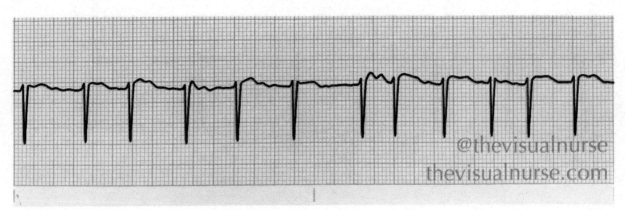

(6 second method)   (Small box method)

RATE: Atrial: _____   Ventricular: _____   Ventricular: _____

RHYTHM: Atrial Regular Irregular   Ventricular Regular Irregular

P WAVES: _____   PR: _____   QRS: _____   QT: _____

ST SEGMENT: Okay Elevated Depressed   T WAVES: _____

28.

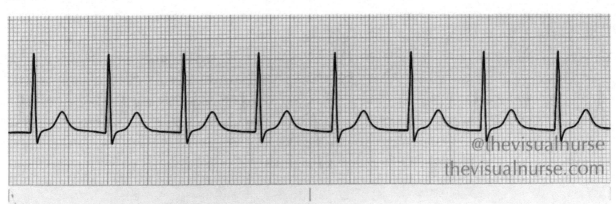

(6 second method)   (Small box method)

RATE: Atrial: _____   Ventricular: _____   Ventricular: _____

RHYTHM: Atrial Regular Irregular   Ventricular Regular Irregular

P WAVES: _____   PR: _____   QRS: _____   QT: _____

ST SEGMENT: Okay Elevated Depressed   T WAVES: _____

29.

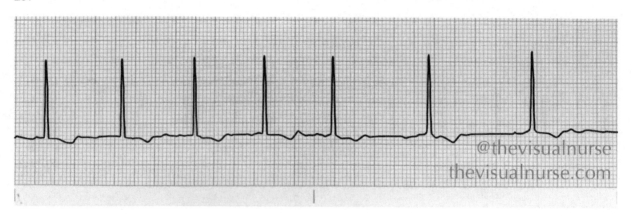

(6 second method)   (Small box method)

RATE: Atrial: _____ Ventricular: _____   Ventricular: _____

RHYTHM: <u>Atrial</u> Regular Irregular   <u>Ventricular</u> Regular Irregular

P WAVES: _____ PR: _____ QRS: _____ QT: _____

ST SEGMENT: Okay Elevated Depressed   T WAVES: _____

30.

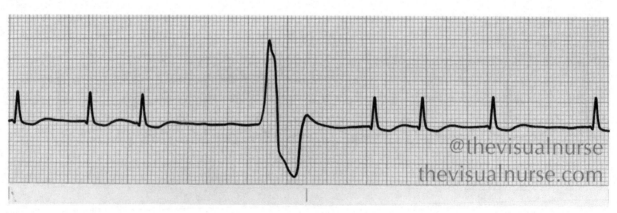

(6 second method)   (Small box method)

RATE: Atrial: _____ Ventricular: _____   Ventricular: _____

RHYTHM: <u>Atrial</u> Regular Irregular   <u>Ventricular</u> Regular Irregular

P WAVES: _____ PR: _____ QRS: _____ QT: _____

ST SEGMENT: Okay Elevated Depressed   T WAVES: _____

31.

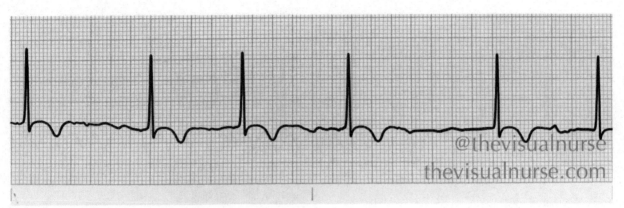

(6 second method)   (Small box method)

RATE: Atrial: _____   Ventricular: _____   Ventricular: _____

RHYTHM: <u>Atrial</u> Regular Irregular   <u>Ventricular</u> Regular Irregular

P WAVES: _____ PR: _____   QRS: _____   QT: _____

ST SEGMENT: Okay Elevated Depressed   T WAVES: _____

32.

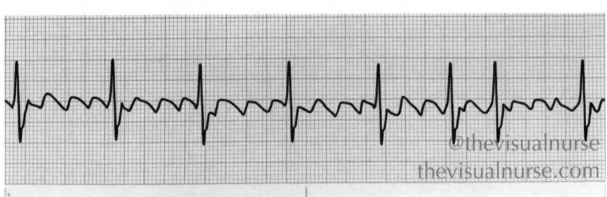

(6 second method)   (Small box method)

RATE: Atrial: _____   Ventricular: _____   Ventricular: _____

RHYTHM: <u>Atrial</u> Regular Irregular   <u>Ventricular</u> Regular Irregular

P WAVES: _____ PR: _____   QRS: _____   QT: _____

ST SEGMENT: Okay Elevated Depressed   T WAVES: _____

33.

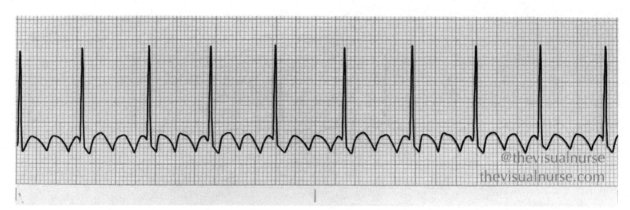

(6 second method) (Small box method)

RATE: Atrial: _____   Ventricular: _____   Ventricular: _____

RHYTHM: <u>Atrial</u> Regular Irregular   <u>Ventricular</u> Regular Irregular

P WAVES: _____ PR: _____   QRS: _____   QT: _____

ST SEGMENT: Okay Elevated Depressed   T WAVES: _____

34.

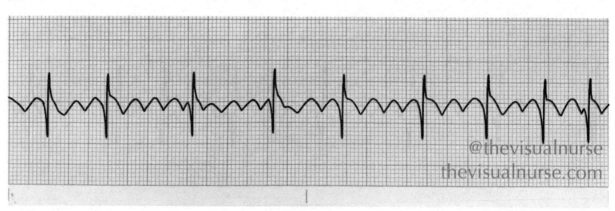

(6 second method) (Small box method)

RATE: Atrial: _____   Ventricular: _____   Ventricular: _____

RHYTHM: <u>Atrial</u> Regular Irregular   <u>Ventricular</u> Regular Irregular

P WAVES: _____ PR: _____   QRS: _____   QT: _____

ST SEGMENT: Okay Elevated Depressed   T WAVES: _____

35.

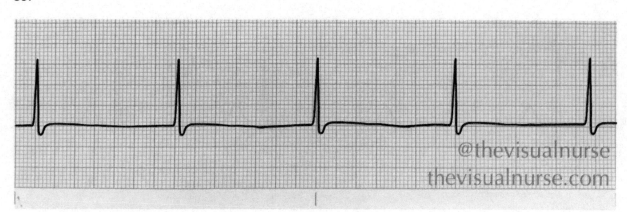

(6 second method)   (Small box method)

RATE: Atrial: _____   Ventricular: _____   Ventricular: _____

RHYTHM: <u>Atrial</u> Regular Irregular   <u>Ventricular</u> Regular Irregular

P WAVES: _____   PR: _____   QRS: _____   QT: _____

ST SEGMENT: Okay Elevated Depressed   T WAVES: _____

36.

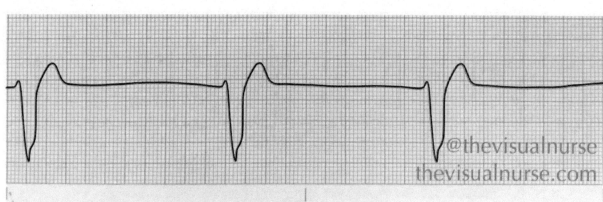

(6 second method)   (Small box method)

RATE: Atrial: _____   Ventricular: _____   Ventricular: _____

RHYTHM: <u>Atrial</u> Regular Irregular   <u>Ventricular</u> Regular Irregular

P WAVES: _____   PR: _____   QRS: _____   QT: _____

ST SEGMENT: Okay Elevated Depressed   T WAVES: _____

37.

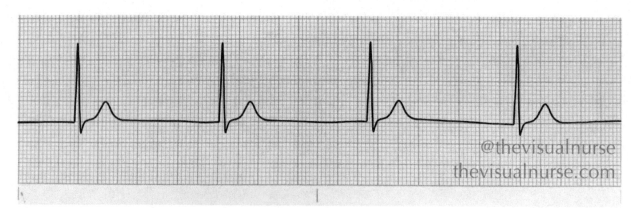

(6 second method)   (Small box method)

RATE: Atrial: _____   Ventricular: _____   Ventricular: _____

RHYTHM: <u>Atrial</u> Regular Irregular   <u>Ventricular</u> Regular Irregular

P WAVES: _____   PR: _____   QRS: _____   QT: _____

ST SEGMENT: Okay Elevated Depressed   T WAVES: _____

38.

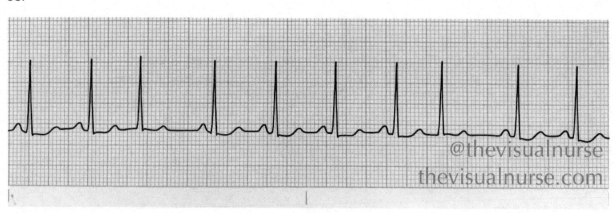

(6 second method)   (Small box method)

RATE: Atrial: _____   Ventricular: _____   Ventricular: _____

RHYTHM: <u>Atrial</u> Regular Irregular   <u>Ventricular</u> Regular Irregular

P WAVES: _____   PR: _____   QRS: _____   QT: _____

ST SEGMENT: Okay Elevated Depressed   T WAVES: _____

39.

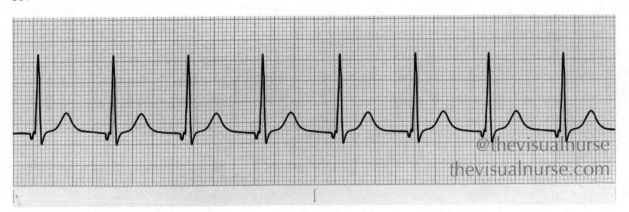

(6 second method)   (Small box method)
RATE: Atrial: _____   Ventricular: _____   Ventricular: _____
RHYTHM: Atrial Regular Irregular   Ventricular Regular Irregular
P WAVES: _____ PR: _____ QRS: _____ QT: _____
ST SEGMENT: Okay Elevated Depressed   T WAVES: _____

40.

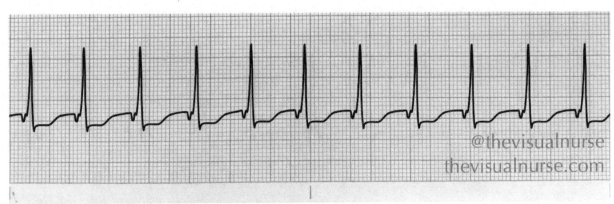

(6 second method)   (Small box method)
RATE: Atrial: _____   Ventricular: _____   Ventricular: _____
RHYTHM: Atrial Regular Irregular   Ventricular Regular Irregular
P WAVES: _____ PR: _____ QRS: _____ QT: _____
ST SEGMENT: Okay Elevated Depressed   T WAVES: _____

41

41.

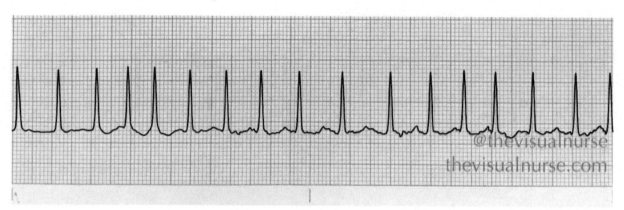

(6 second method)   (Small box method)

RATE: Atrial: _____   Ventricular: _____   Ventricular: _____

RHYTHM: <u>Atrial</u> Regular Irregular   <u>Ventricular</u> Regular Irregular

P WAVES: _____   PR: _____   QRS: _____   QT: _____

ST SEGMENT: Okay Elevated Depressed   T WAVES: _____

42.

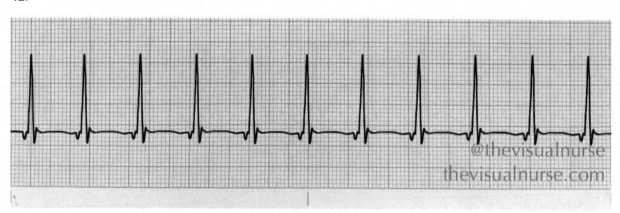

(6 second method)   (Small box method)

RATE: Atrial: _____   Ventricular: _____   Ventricular: _____

RHYTHM: <u>Atrial</u> Regular Irregular   <u>Ventricular</u> Regular Irregular

P WAVES: _____   PR: _____   QRS: _____   QT: _____

ST SEGMENT: Okay Elevated Depressed   T WAVES: _____

43.

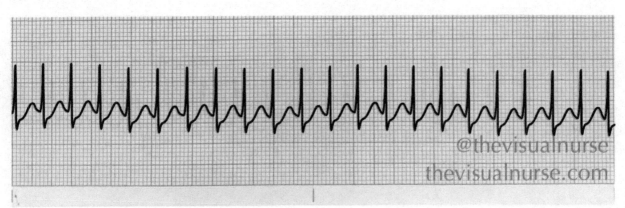

(6 second method) (Small box method)

RATE: Atrial: _____ Ventricular: _____ Ventricular: _____

RHYTHM: <u>Atrial</u> Regular Irregular <u>Ventricular</u> Regular Irregular

P WAVES: _____ PR: _____ QRS: _____ QT: _____

ST SEGMENT: Okay Elevated Depressed T WAVES: _____

44.

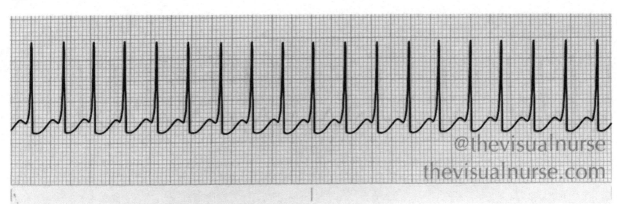

(6 second method) (Small box method)

RATE: Atrial: _____ Ventricular: _____ Ventricular: _____

RHYTHM: <u>Atrial</u> Regular Irregular <u>Ventricular</u> Regular Irregular

P WAVES: _____ PR: _____ QRS: _____ QT: _____

ST SEGMENT: Okay Elevated Depressed T WAVES: _____

45.

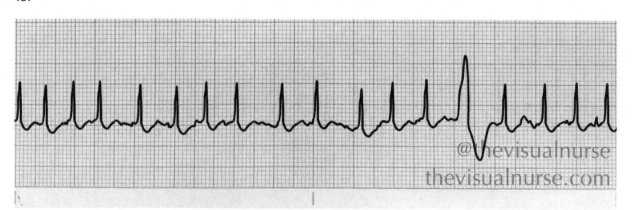

(6 second method)   (Small box method)

RATE: Atrial: _____   Ventricular: _____   Ventricular: _____

RHYTHM: <u>Atrial</u> Regular Irregular   <u>Ventricular</u> Regular Irregular

P WAVES: _____   PR: _____   QRS: _____   QT: _____

ST SEGMENT: Okay Elevated Depressed   T WAVES: _____

46.

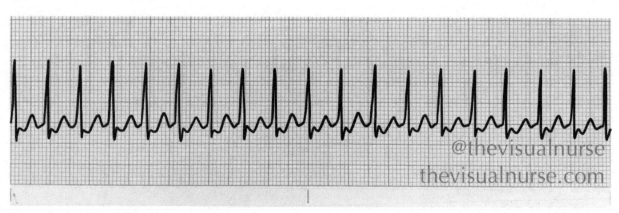

(6 second method)   (Small box method)

RATE: Atrial: _____   Ventricular: _____   Ventricular: _____

RHYTHM: <u>Atrial</u> Regular Irregular   <u>Ventricular</u> Regular Irregular

P WAVES: _____   PR: _____   QRS: _____   QT: _____

ST SEGMENT: Okay Elevated Depressed   T WAVES: _____

47.

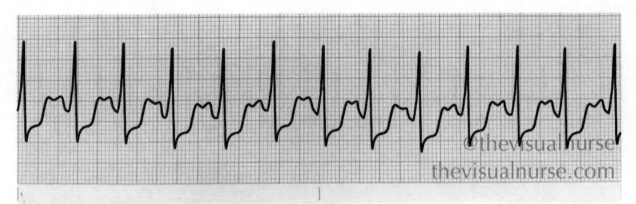

(6 second method)   (Small box method)
RATE: Atrial: _____   Ventricular: _____   Ventricular: _____
RHYTHM: <u>Atrial</u> Regular Irregular   <u>Ventricular</u> Regular Irregular
P WAVES: _____   PR: _____   QRS: _____   QT: _____
ST SEGMENT: Okay Elevated Depressed   T WAVES: _____

48.

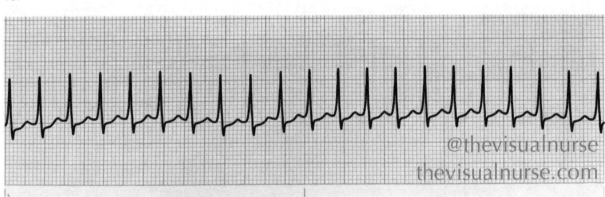

(6 second method)   (Small box method)
RATE: Atrial: _____   Ventricular: _____   Ventricular: _____
RHYTHM: <u>Atrial</u> Regular Irregular   <u>Ventricular</u> Regular Irregular
P WAVES: _____   PR: _____   QRS: _____   QT: _____
ST SEGMENT: Okay Elevated Depressed   T WAVES: _____

49.

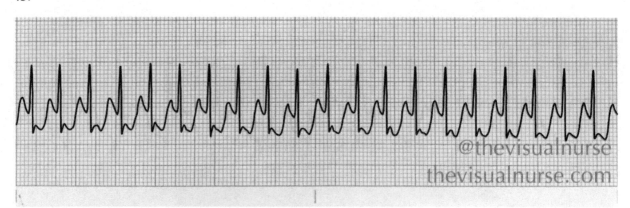

(6 second method)   (Small box method)

RATE: Atrial: _____   Ventricular: _____   Ventricular: _____

RHYTHM: <u>Atrial</u> Regular Irregular   <u>Ventricular</u> Regular Irregular

P WAVES: _____   PR: _____   QRS: _____   QT: _____

ST SEGMENT: Okay Elevated Depressed   T WAVES: _____

50.

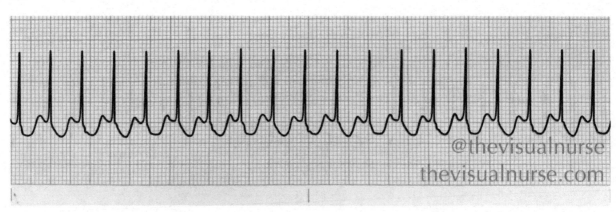

(6 second method)   (Small box method)

RATE: Atrial: _____   Ventricular: _____   Ventricular: _____

RHYTHM: <u>Atrial</u> Regular Irregular   <u>Ventricular</u> Regular Irregular

P WAVES: _____   PR: _____   QRS: _____   QT: _____

ST SEGMENT: Okay Elevated Depressed   T WAVES: _____

51.

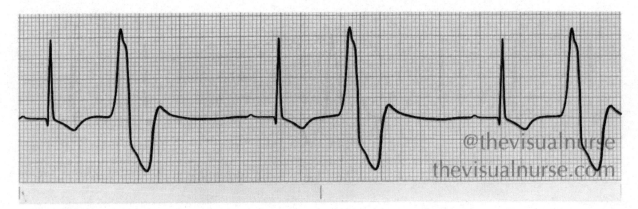

(6 second method)   (Small box method)

RATE: Atrial: _____   Ventricular: _____   Ventricular: _____

RHYTHM: <u>Atrial</u> Regular Irregular   <u>Ventricular</u> Regular Irregular

P WAVES: _____   PR: _____   QRS: _____   QT: _____

ST SEGMENT: Okay Elevated Depressed   T WAVES: _____

52.

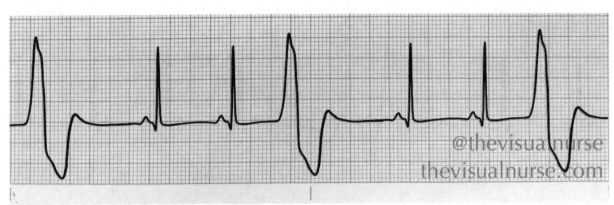

(6 second method)   (Small box method)

RATE: Atrial: _____   Ventricular: _____   Ventricular: _____

RHYTHM: <u>Atrial</u> Regular Irregular   <u>Ventricular</u> Regular Irregular

P WAVES: _____   PR: _____   QRS: _____   QT: _____

ST SEGMENT: Okay Elevated Depressed   T WAVES: _____

53.

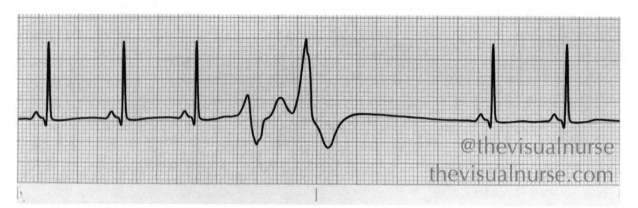

(6 second method)   (Small box method)

RATE: Atrial: _____   Ventricular: _____   Ventricular: _____

RHYTHM: <u>Atrial</u> Regular Irregular   Ventricular Regular Irregular

P WAVES: _____ PR: _____ QRS: _____ QT: _____

ST SEGMENT: Okay Elevated Depressed   T WAVES: _____

54.

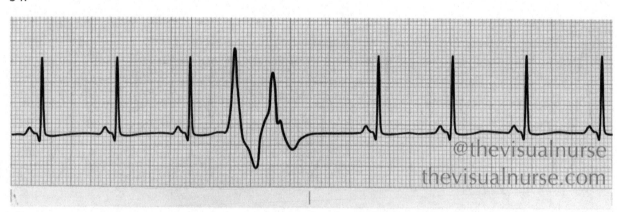

(6 second method)   (Small box method)

RATE: Atrial: _____   Ventricular: _____   Ventricular: _____

RHYTHM: <u>Atrial</u> Regular Irregular   Ventricular Regular Irregular

P WAVES: _____ PR: _____ QRS: _____ QT: _____

ST SEGMENT: Okay Elevated Depressed   T WAVES: _____

55.

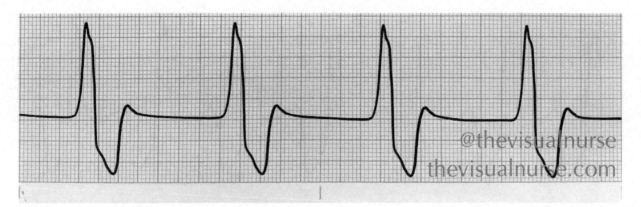

(6 second method)   (Small box method)
RATE: Atrial: _____   Ventricular: _____   Ventricular: _____
RHYTHM: <u>Atrial</u> Regular Irregular   <u>Ventricular</u> Regular Irregular
P WAVES: _____ PR: _____   QRS: _____ QT: _____
ST SEGMENT: Okay Elevated Depressed   T WAVES: _____

56.

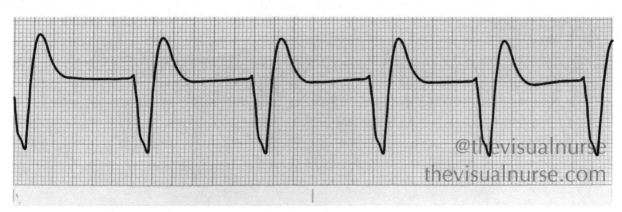

(6 second method)   (Small box method)
RATE: Atrial: _____   Ventricular: _____   Ventricular: _____
RHYTHM: <u>Atrial</u> Regular Irregular   <u>Ventricular</u> Regular Irregular
P WAVES: _____ PR: _____   QRS: _____ QT: _____
ST SEGMENT: Okay Elevated Depressed   T WAVES: _____

57.

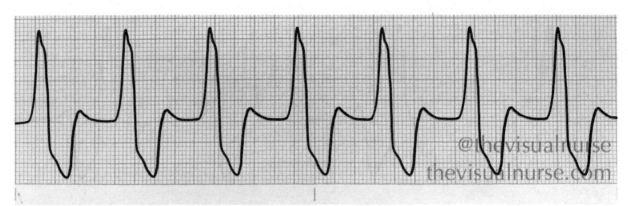

            (6 second method)   (Small box method)

RATE: Atrial: _____ Ventricular: _____   Ventricular: _____

RHYTHM: <u>Atrial</u> Regular Irregular   <u>Ventricular</u> Regular Irregular

P WAVES: _____ PR: _____ QRS: _____ QT: _____

ST SEGMENT: Okay Elevated Depressed   T WAVES: _____

58.

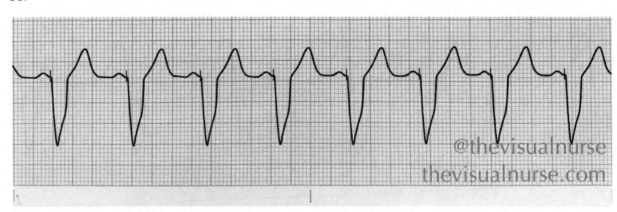

            (6 second method)   (Small box method)

RATE: Atrial: _____ Ventricular: _____   Ventricular: _____

RHYTHM: <u>Atrial</u> Regular Irregular   <u>Ventricular</u> Regular Irregular

P WAVES: _____ PR: _____ QRS: _____ QT: _____

ST SEGMENT: Okay Elevated Depressed   T WAVES: _____

59.

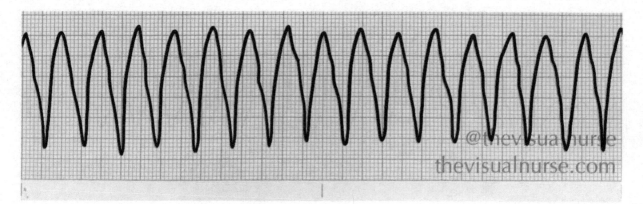

(6 second method)   (Small box method)

RATE: Atrial: _____   Ventricular: _____   Ventricular: _____

RHYTHM: <u>Atrial</u> Regular Irregular   <u>Ventricular</u> Regular Irregular

P WAVES: _____   PR: _____   QRS: _____   QT: _____

ST SEGMENT: Okay Elevated Depressed   T WAVES: _____

60.

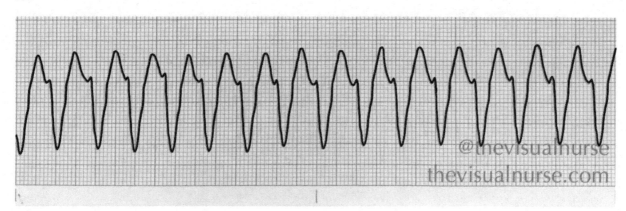

(6 second method)   (Small box method)

RATE: Atrial: _____   Ventricular: _____   Ventricular: _____

RHYTHM: <u>Atrial</u> Regular Irregular   <u>Ventricular</u> Regular Irregular

P WAVES: _____   PR: _____   QRS: _____   QT: _____

ST SEGMENT: Okay Elevated Depressed   T WAVES: _____

61.

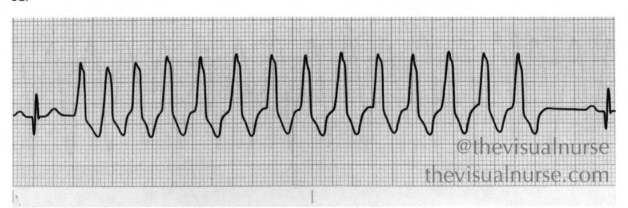

(6 second method)   (Small box method)

RATE: Atrial: _____   Ventricular: _____   Ventricular: _____

RHYTHM: <u>Atrial</u> Regular Irregular   <u>Ventricular</u> Regular Irregular

P WAVES: _____   PR: _____   QRS: _____   QT: _____

ST SEGMENT: Okay Elevated Depressed   T WAVES: _____

62.

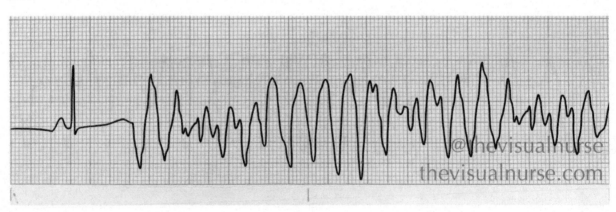

(6 second method)   (Small box method)

RATE: Atrial: _____   Ventricular: _____   Ventricular: _____

RHYTHM: <u>Atrial</u> Regular Irregular   <u>Ventricular</u> Regular Irregular

P WAVES: _____   PR: _____   QRS: _____   QT: _____

ST SEGMENT: Okay Elevated Depressed   T WAVES: _____

63.

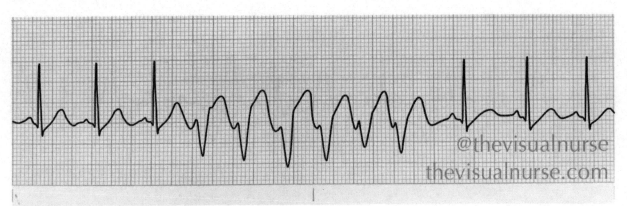

(6 second method)   (Small box method)

RATE: Atrial: _____   Ventricular: _____   Ventricular: _____

RHYTHM: <u>Atrial</u> Regular Irregular   <u>Ventricular</u> Regular Irregular

P WAVES: _____ PR: _____ QRS: _____ QT: _____

ST SEGMENT: Okay Elevated Depressed   T WAVES: _____

64.

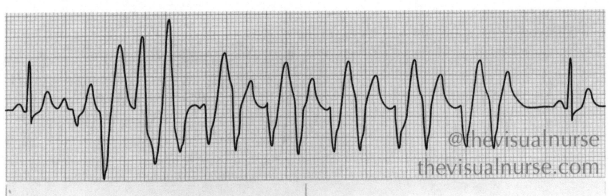

(6 second method)   (Small box method)

RATE: Atrial: _____   Ventricular: _____   Ventricular: _____

RHYTHM: <u>Atrial</u> Regular Irregular   <u>Ventricular</u> Regular Irregular

P WAVES: _____ PR: _____ QRS: _____ QT: _____

ST SEGMENT: Okay Elevated Depressed   T WAVES: _____

55

65.

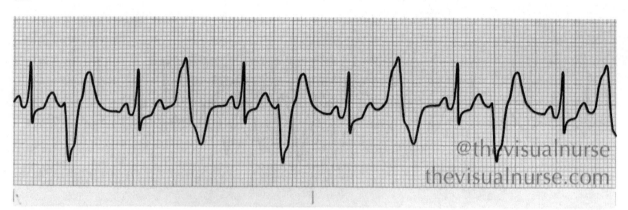

(6 second method)   (Small box method)
RATE: Atrial: _____   Ventricular: _____   Ventricular: _____
RHYTHM: <u>Atrial</u> Regular Irregular   <u>Ventricular</u> Regular Irregular
P WAVES: _____   PR: _____   QRS: _____   QT: _____
ST SEGMENT: Okay Elevated Depressed   T WAVES: _____

66.

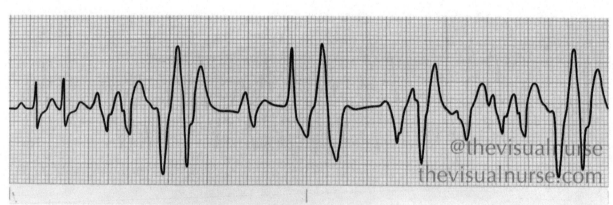

(6 second method)   (Small box method)
RATE: Atrial: _____   Ventricular: _____   Ventricular: _____
RHYTHM: <u>Atrial</u> Regular Irregular   <u>Ventricular</u> Regular Irregular
P WAVES: _____   PR: _____   QRS: _____   QT: _____
ST SEGMENT: Okay Elevated Depressed   T WAVES: _____

67.

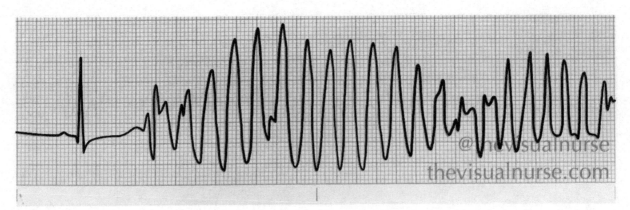

(6 second method)   (Small box method)

RATE: Atrial: _____   Ventricular: _____   Ventricular: _____

RHYTHM: <u>Atrial</u> Regular Irregular   <u>Ventricular</u> Regular Irregular

P WAVES: _____ PR: _____ QRS: _____ QT: _____

ST SEGMENT: Okay Elevated Depressed   T WAVES: _____

68.

(6 second method)   (Small box method)

RATE: Atrial: _____   Ventricular: _____   Ventricular: _____

RHYTHM: <u>Atrial</u> Regular Irregular   <u>Ventricular</u> Regular Irregular

P WAVES: _____ PR: _____ QRS: _____ QT: _____

ST SEGMENT: Okay Elevated Depressed   T WAVES: _____

69.

(6 second method)   (Small box method)

RATE: Atrial: _____ Ventricular: _____   Ventricular: _____

RHYTHM: <u>Atrial</u> Regular Irregular   <u>Ventricular</u> Regular Irregular

P WAVES: _____ PR: _____ QRS: _____ QT: _____

ST SEGMENT: Okay Elevated Depressed   T WAVES: _____

70.

(6 second method)   (Small box method)

RATE: Atrial: _____ Ventricular: _____   Ventricular: _____

RHYTHM: <u>Atrial</u> Regular Irregular   <u>Ventricular</u> Regular Irregular

P WAVES: _____ PR: _____ QRS: _____ QT: _____

ST SEGMENT: Okay Elevated Depressed   T WAVES: _____

71.

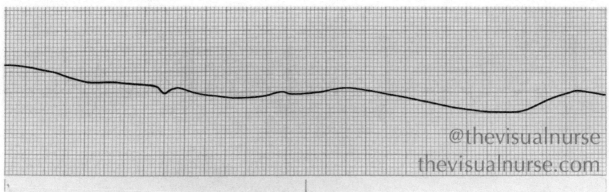

(6 second method)   (Small box method)

RATE: Atrial: _____   Ventricular: _____   Ventricular: _____

RHYTHM: <u>Atrial</u> Regular Irregular   <u>Ventricular</u> Regular Irregular

P WAVES: _____ PR: _____ QRS: _____ QT: _____

ST SEGMENT: Okay Elevated Depressed   T WAVES: _____

72.

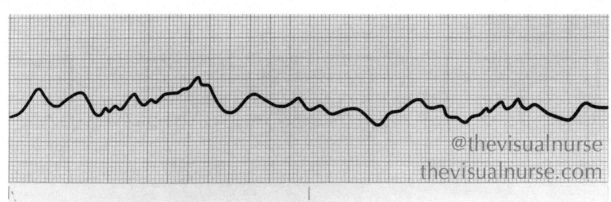

(6 second method)   (Small box method)

RATE: Atrial: _____   Ventricular: _____   Ventricular: _____

RHYTHM: <u>Atrial</u> Regular Irregular   <u>Ventricular</u> Regular Irregular

P WAVES: _____ PR: _____ QRS: _____ QT: _____

ST SEGMENT: Okay Elevated Depressed   T WAVES: _____

73.

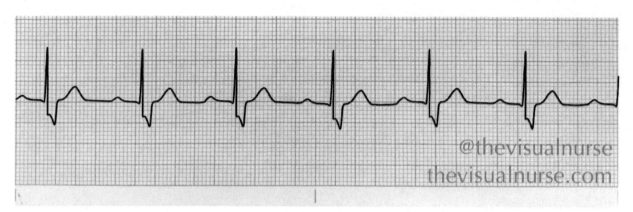

(6 second method)   (Small box method)
RATE: Atrial: _____   Ventricular: _____   Ventricular: _____
RHYTHM: <u>Atrial</u> Regular Irregular   <u>Ventricular</u> Regular Irregular
P WAVES: _____ PR: _____   QRS: _____ QT: _____
ST SEGMENT: Okay Elevated Depressed   T WAVES: _____

74.

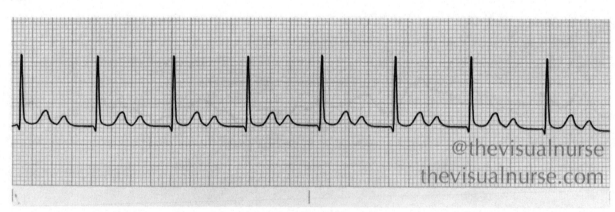

(6 second method)   (Small box method)
RATE: Atrial: _____   Ventricular: _____   Ventricular: _____
RHYTHM: <u>Atrial</u> Regular Irregular   <u>Ventricular</u> Regular Irregular
P WAVES: _____ PR: _____   QRS: _____ QT: _____
ST SEGMENT: Okay Elevated Depressed   T WAVES: _____

75.

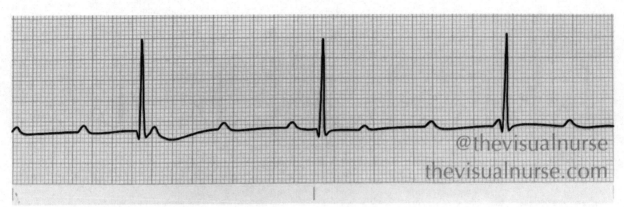

        (6 second method)   (Small box method)

RATE: Atrial: _____   Ventricular: _____   Ventricular: _____

RHYTHM: <u>Atrial</u> Regular Irregular   <u>Ventricular</u> Regular Irregular

P WAVES: _____   PR: _____   QRS: _____   QT: _____

ST SEGMENT: Okay Elevated Depressed   T WAVES: _____

76.

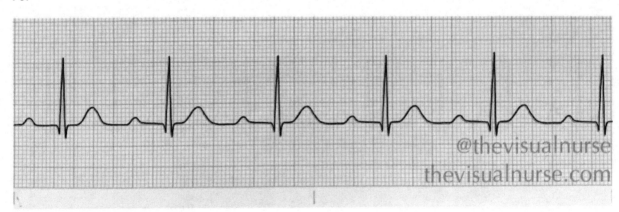

        (6 second method)   (Small box method)

RATE: Atrial: _____   Ventricular: _____   Ventricular: _____

RHYTHM: <u>Atrial</u> Regular Irregular   <u>Ventricular</u> Regular Irregular

P WAVES: _____   PR: _____   QRS: _____   QT: _____

ST SEGMENT: Okay Elevated Depressed   T WAVES: _____

77.

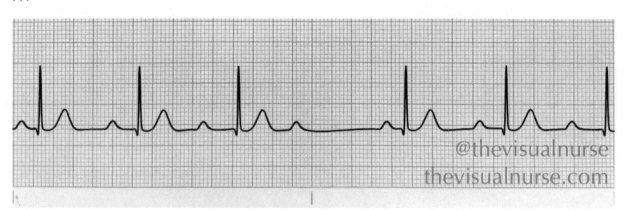

(6 second method)   (Small box method)

RATE: Atrial: _____ Ventricular: _____   Ventricular: _____

RHYTHM: <u>Atrial</u> Regular Irregular   <u>Ventricular</u> Regular Irregular

P WAVES: _____ PR: _____ QRS: _____ QT: _____

ST SEGMENT: Okay Elevated Depressed   T WAVES: _____

78.

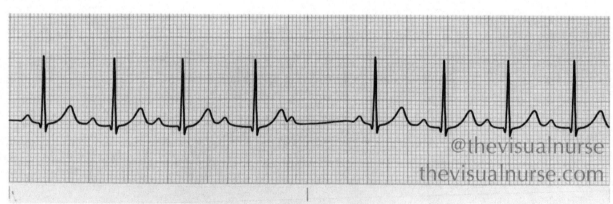

(6 second method)   (Small box method)

RATE: Atrial: _____ Ventricular: _____   Ventricular: _____

RHYTHM: <u>Atrial</u> Regular Irregular   <u>Ventricular</u> Regular Irregular

P WAVES: _____ PR: _____ QRS: _____ QT: _____

ST SEGMENT: Okay Elevated Depressed   T WAVES: _____

79.

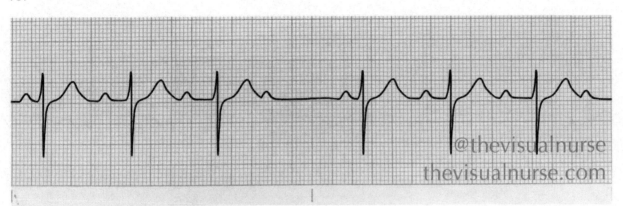

(6 second method)   (Small box method)

RATE: Atrial: _____ Ventricular: _____   Ventricular: _____

RHYTHM: <u>Atrial</u> Regular Irregular   <u>Ventricular</u> Regular Irregular

P WAVES: _____ PR: _____ QRS: _____ QT: _____

ST SEGMENT: Okay Elevated Depressed   T WAVES: _____

80.

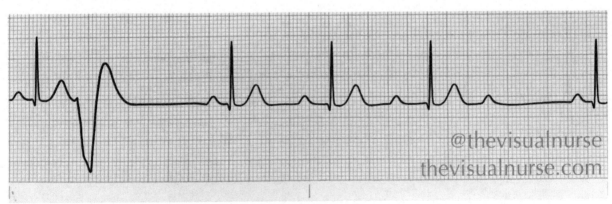

(6 second method)   (Small box method)

RATE: Atrial: _____ Ventricular: _____   Ventricular: _____

RHYTHM: <u>Atrial</u> Regular Irregular   <u>Ventricular</u> Regular Irregular

P WAVES: _____ PR: _____ QRS: _____ QT: _____

ST SEGMENT: Okay Elevated Depressed   T WAVES: _____

81.

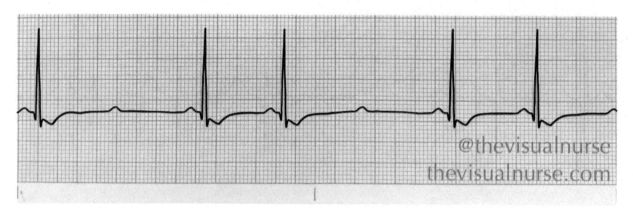

(6 second method)   (Small box method)
RATE: Atrial: _____   Ventricular: _____   Ventricular: _____
RHYTHM: Atrial Regular Irregular   Ventricular Regular Irregular
P WAVES: _____   PR: _____   QRS: _____   QT: _____
ST SEGMENT: Okay Elevated Depressed   T WAVES: _____

82.

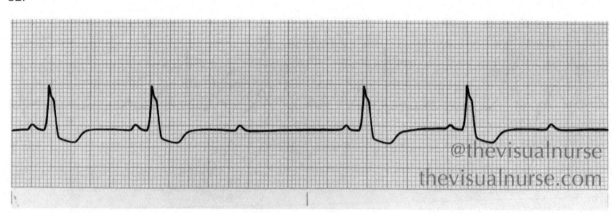

(6 second method)   (Small box method)
RATE: Atrial: _____   Ventricular: _____   Ventricular: _____
RHYTHM: Atrial Regular Irregular   Ventricular Regular Irregular
P WAVES: _____   PR: _____   QRS: _____   QT: _____
ST SEGMENT: Okay Elevated Depressed   T WAVES: _____

83.

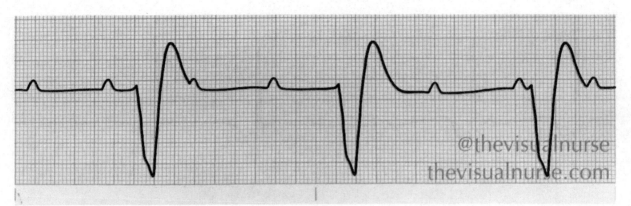

(6 second method)   (Small box method)

RATE: Atrial:_____ Ventricular:_____   Ventricular:_____

RHYTHM: <u>Atrial</u> Regular Irregular   <u>Ventricular</u> Regular Irregular

P WAVES:_____ PR:_____ QRS:_____ QT:_____

ST SEGMENT: Okay Elevated Depressed   T WAVES:_____

84.

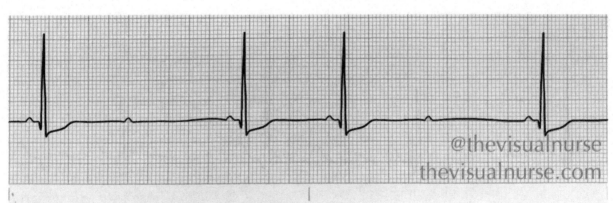

(6 second method)   (Small box method)

RATE: Atrial:_____ Ventricular:_____   Ventricular:_____

RHYTHM: <u>Atrial</u> Regular Irregular   <u>Ventricular</u> Regular Irregular

P WAVES:_____ PR:_____ QRS:_____ QT:_____

ST SEGMENT: Okay Elevated Depressed   T WAVES:_____

85.

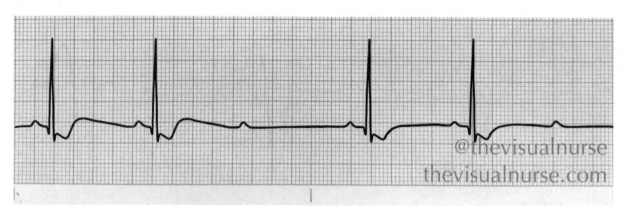

(6 second method)   (Small box method)

RATE: Atrial: _____   Ventricular: _____   Ventricular: _____

RHYTHM: <u>Atrial</u> Regular Irregular   <u>Ventricular</u> Regular Irregular

P WAVES: _____ PR: _____ QRS: _____ QT: _____

ST SEGMENT: Okay Elevated Depressed   T WAVES: _____

86.

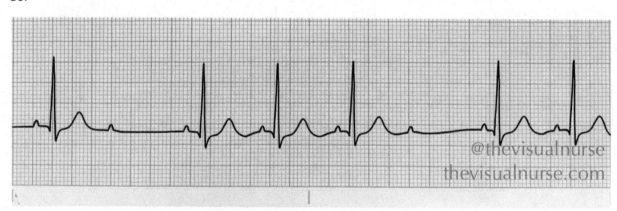

(6 second method)   (Small box method)

RATE: Atrial: _____   Ventricular: _____   Ventricular: _____

RHYTHM: <u>Atrial</u> Regular Irregular   <u>Ventricular</u> Regular Irregular

P WAVES: _____ PR: _____ QRS: _____ QT: _____

ST SEGMENT: Okay Elevated Depressed   T WAVES: _____

87.

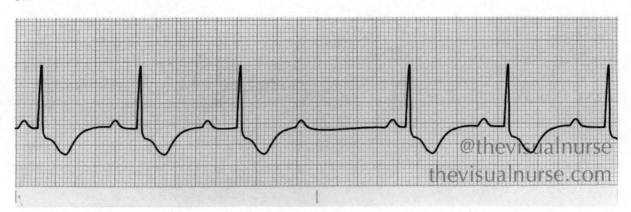

(6 second method)   (Small box method)

RATE: Atrial: _____ Ventricular: _____   Ventricular: _____

RHYTHM: <u>Atrial</u> Regular Irregular   <u>Ventricular</u> Regular Irregular

P WAVES: _____ PR: _____ QRS: _____ QT: _____

ST SEGMENT: Okay Elevated Depressed   T WAVES: _____

88.

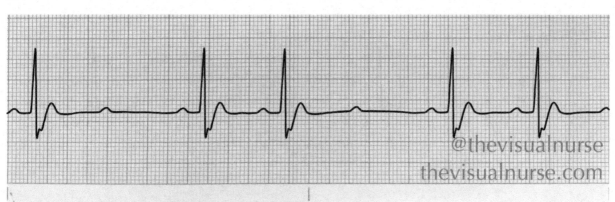

(6 second method)   (Small box method)

RATE: Atrial: _____ Ventricular: _____   Ventricular: _____

RHYTHM: <u>Atrial</u> Regular Irregular   <u>Ventricular</u> Regular Irregular

P WAVES: _____ PR: _____ QRS: _____ QT: _____

ST SEGMENT: Okay Elevated Depressed   T WAVES: _____

89.

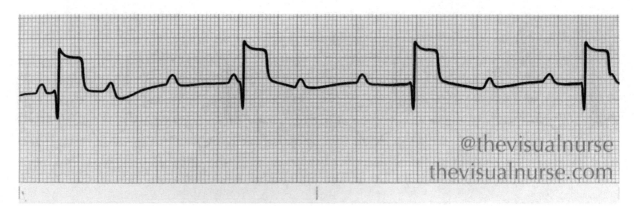

(6 second method)   (Small box method)

RATE: Atrial: _____ Ventricular: _____   Ventricular: _____

RHYTHM: <u>Atrial</u> Regular Irregular   <u>Ventricular</u> Regular Irregular

P WAVES: _____ PR: _____ QRS: _____ QT: _____

ST SEGMENT: Okay Elevated Depressed   T WAVES: _____

90.

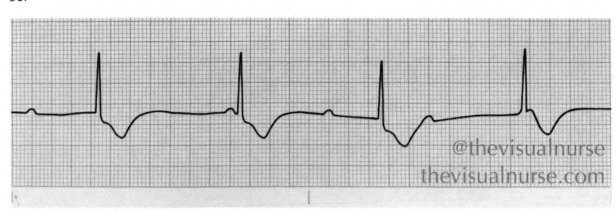

(6 second method)   (Small box method)

RATE: Atrial: _____ Ventricular: _____   Ventricular: _____

RHYTHM: <u>Atrial</u> Regular Irregular   <u>Ventricular</u> Regular Irregular

P WAVES: _____ PR: _____ QRS: _____ QT: _____

ST SEGMENT: Okay Elevated Depressed   T WAVES: _____

91.

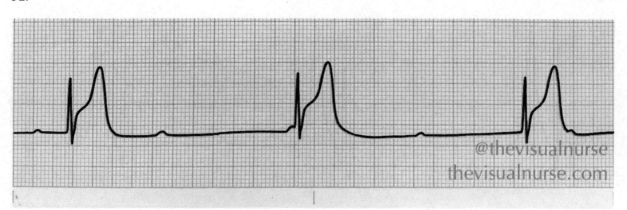

(6 second method)   (Small box method)

RATE: Atrial: _____ Ventricular: _____   Ventricular: _____

RHYTHM: <u>Atrial</u> Regular Irregular   <u>Ventricular</u> Regular Irregular

P WAVES: _____ PR: _____ QRS: _____ QT: _____

ST SEGMENT: Okay Elevated Depressed   T WAVES: _____

92.

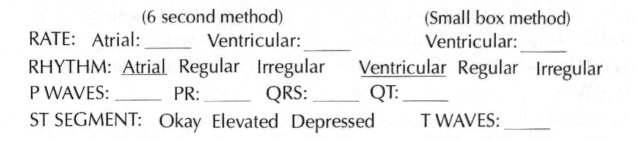
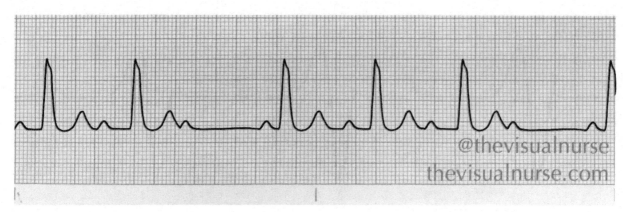

(6 second method)   (Small box method)

RATE: Atrial: _____ Ventricular: _____   Ventricular: _____

RHYTHM: <u>Atrial</u> Regular Irregular   <u>Ventricular</u> Regular Irregular

P WAVES: _____ PR: _____ QRS: _____ QT: _____

ST SEGMENT: Okay Elevated Depressed   T WAVES: _____

93.

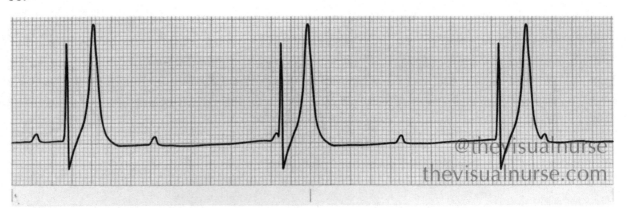

(6 second method)   (Small box method)
RATE: Atrial: _____ Ventricular: _____   Ventricular: _____
RHYTHM: <u>Atrial</u> Regular Irregular   <u>Ventricular</u> Regular Irregular
P WAVES: _____ PR: _____ QRS: _____ QT: _____
ST SEGMENT: Okay Elevated Depressed   T WAVES: _____

94.

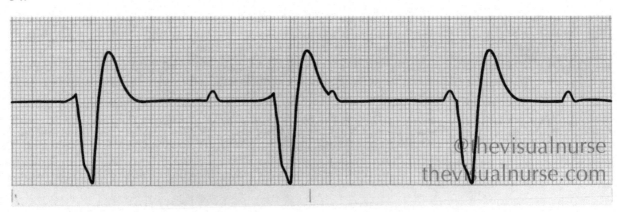

(6 second method)   (Small box method)
RATE: Atrial: _____ Ventricular: _____   Ventricular: _____
RHYTHM: <u>Atrial</u> Regular Irregular   <u>Ventricular</u> Regular Irregular
P WAVES: _____ PR: _____ QRS: _____ QT: _____
ST SEGMENT: Okay Elevated Depressed   T WAVES: _____

95.

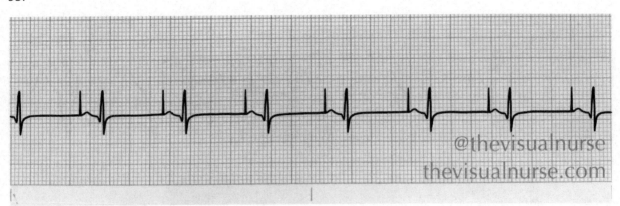

(6 second method)   (Small box method)

RATE: Atrial: _____ Ventricular: _____   Ventricular: _____

RHYTHM: <u>Atrial</u> Regular Irregular   <u>Ventricular</u> Regular Irregular

P WAVES: _____ PR: _____ QRS: _____ QT: _____

ST SEGMENT: Okay Elevated Depressed   T WAVES: _____

96.

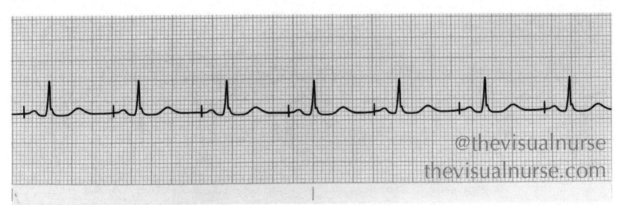

(6 second method)   (Small box method)

RATE: Atrial: _____ Ventricular: _____   Ventricular: _____

RHYTHM: <u>Atrial</u> Regular Irregular   <u>Ventricular</u> Regular Irregular

P WAVES: _____ PR: _____ QRS: _____ QT: _____

ST SEGMENT: Okay Elevated Depressed   T WAVES: _____

97.

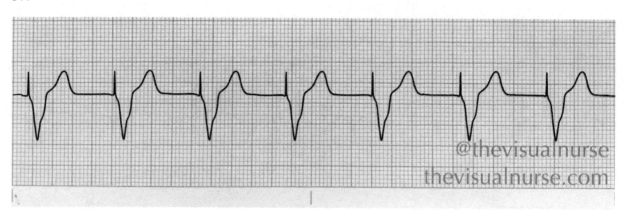

(6 second method)   (Small box method)

RATE: Atrial: _____ Ventricular: _____   Ventricular: _____

RHYTHM: <u>Atrial</u> Regular Irregular   <u>Ventricular</u> Regular Irregular

P WAVES: _____ PR: _____ QRS: _____ QT: _____

ST SEGMENT: Okay Elevated Depressed   T WAVES: _____

98.

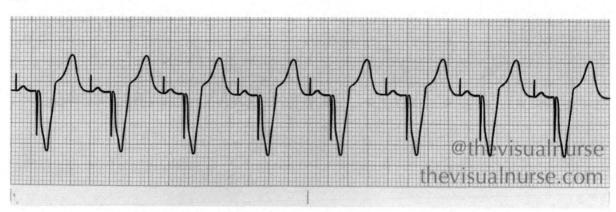

(6 second method)   (Small box method)

RATE: Atrial: _____ Ventricular: _____   Ventricular: _____

RHYTHM: <u>Atrial</u> Regular Irregular   <u>Ventricular</u> Regular Irregular

P WAVES: _____ PR: _____ QRS: _____ QT: _____

ST SEGMENT: Okay Elevated Depressed   T WAVES: _____

99.

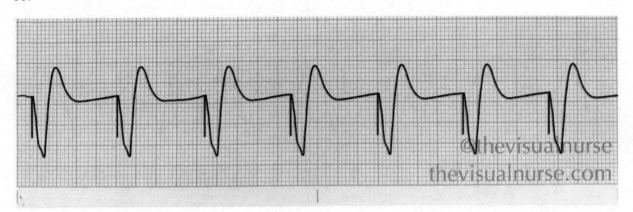

(6 second method)   (Small box method)

RATE: Atrial: _____ Ventricular: _____   Ventricular: _____

RHYTHM: <u>Atrial</u> Regular Irregular   <u>Ventricular</u> Regular Irregular

P WAVES: _____   PR: _____   QRS: _____   QT: _____

ST SEGMENT: Okay Elevated Depressed   T WAVES: _____

100.

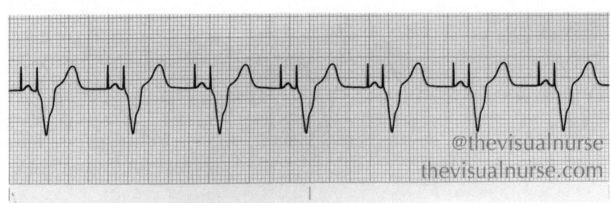

(6 second method)   (Small box method)

RATE: Atrial: _____ Ventricular: _____   Ventricular: _____

RHYTHM: <u>Atrial</u> Regular Irregular   <u>Ventricular</u> Regular Irregular

P WAVES: _____   PR: _____   QRS: _____   QT: _____

ST SEGMENT: Okay Elevated Depressed   T WAVES: _____

101.

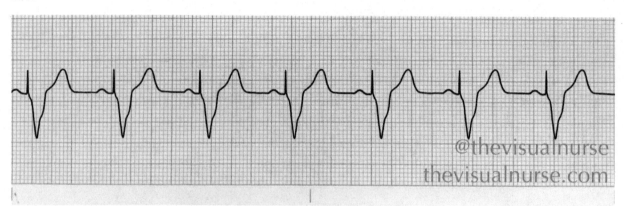

(6 second method)   (Small box method)

RATE: Atrial: _____   Ventricular: _____   Ventricular: _____

RHYTHM: <u>Atrial</u> Regular Irregular   <u>Ventricular</u> Regular Irregular

P WAVES: _____   PR: _____   QRS: _____   QT: _____

ST SEGMENT: Okay Elevated Depressed   T WAVES: _____

102.

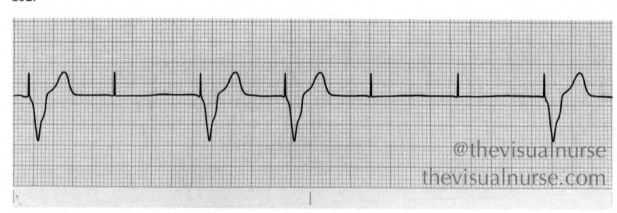

(6 second method)   (Small box method)

RATE: Atrial: _____   Ventricular: _____   Ventricular: _____

RHYTHM: <u>Atrial</u> Regular Irregular   <u>Ventricular</u> Regular Irregular

P WAVES: _____   PR: _____   QRS: _____   QT: _____

ST SEGMENT: Okay Elevated Depressed   T WAVES: _____

103.

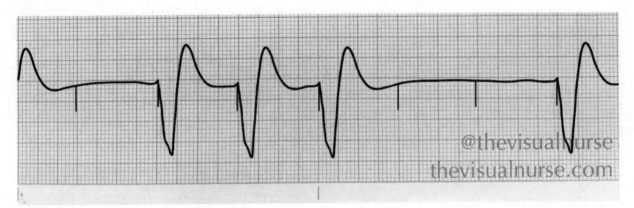

(6 second method)   (Small box method)
RATE: Atrial: _____   Ventricular: _____   Ventricular: _____
RHYTHM: <u>Atrial</u> Regular Irregular   <u>Ventricular</u> Regular Irregular
P WAVES: _____   PR: _____   QRS: _____   QT: _____
ST SEGMENT: Okay Elevated Depressed   T WAVES: _____

104.

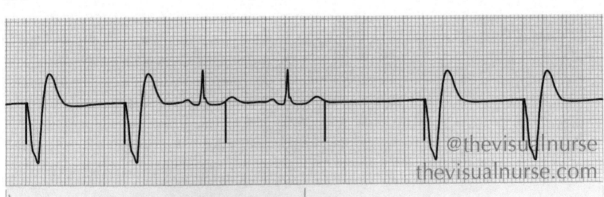

(6 second method)   (Small box method)
RATE: Atrial: _____   Ventricular: _____   Ventricular: _____
RHYTHM: <u>Atrial</u> Regular Irregular   <u>Ventricular</u> Regular Irregular
P WAVES: _____   PR: _____   QRS: _____   QT: _____
ST SEGMENT: Okay Elevated Depressed   T WAVES: _____

105.

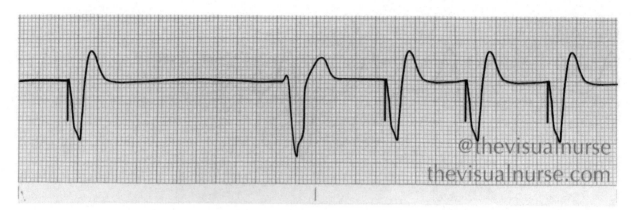

(6 second method) (Small box method)

RATE: Atrial: _____   Ventricular: _____   Ventricular: _____

RHYTHM: <u>Atrial</u> Regular Irregular   <u>Ventricular</u> Regular Irregular

P WAVES: _____   PR: _____   QRS: _____   QT: _____

ST SEGMENT: Okay Elevated Depressed   T WAVES: _____

ANSWER KEYS

1.

Normal sinus rhythm

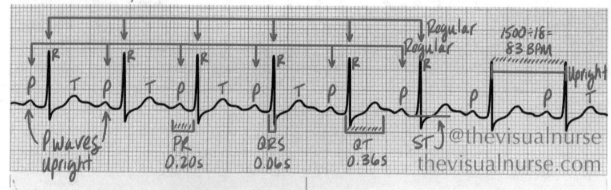

(6 second method)

RATE: Atrial: 80 Ventricular: 80

(Small box method)

Ventricular: 83

RHYTHM: Atrial (Regular) Irregular Ventricular (Regular) Irregular

P WAVES: Upright PR: 0.20s QRS: 0.06s QT: 0.36s

ST SEGMENT: (Okay) Elevated Depressed T WAVES: Upright

2.

Sinus rhythm with wide QRS & downsloping ST depression

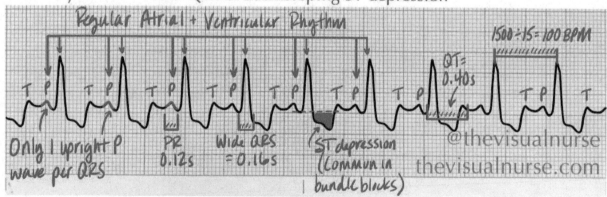

(6 second method)

RATE: Atrial: 90 Ventricular: 90

(Small box method)

Ventricular: 100

RHYTHM: Atrial (Regular) Irregular Ventricular (Regular) Irregular

P WAVES: Upright PR: 0.12s QRS: 0.16s QT: 0.40s

ST SEGMENT: Okay Elevated (Depressed) T WAVES: Biphasic

3.

Sinus rhythm with "tombstoning" ST elevation

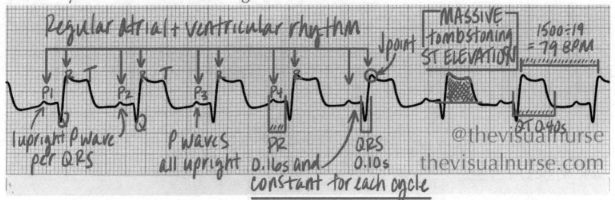

(6 second method) (Small box method)

RATE: Atrial: __80__ Ventricular: __80__ Ventricular: __79__

RHYTHM: Atrial (Regular) Irregular   Ventricular (Regular) Irregular

P WAVES: Upright PR: 0.16s QRS: 0.10s QT: 0.40s

ST SEGMENT: Okay (Elevated) Depressed   T WAVES: Upright

4.

Sinus tachycardia with a wide QRS and ventricular couplet

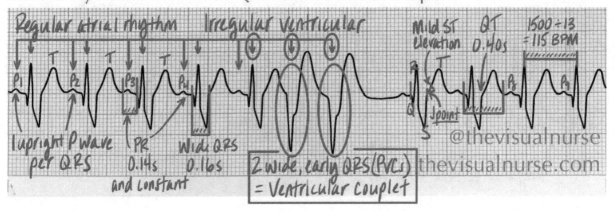

(6 second method) (Small box method)

RATE: Atrial: __90__ Ventricular: __90__ Ventricular: __115__

RHYTHM: Atrial (Regular) Irregular   Ventricular Regular (Irregular)

P WAVES: Upright PR: 0.14s QRS: 0.16s QT: 0.40s

ST SEGMENT: Okay (Elevated) Depressed   T WAVES: Upright

5.

Sinus rhythm with flat T waves

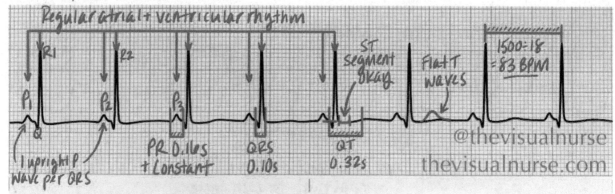

(6 second method) (Small box method)

RATE: Atrial: _80_ Ventricular: _80_ Ventricular: _83_

RHYTHM: Atrial (Regular) Irregular Ventricular (Regular) Irregular

P WAVES: Upright PR: 0.16s QRS: 0.10s QT: 0.32s

ST SEGMENT: (Okay) Elevated Depressed T WAVES: Flat

6.

Sinus tachycardia

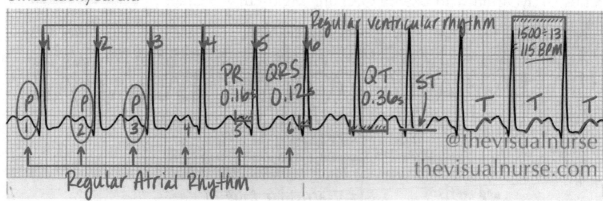

(6 second method) (Small box method)

RATE: Atrial: _110_ Ventricular: _110_ Ventricular: 115

RHYTHM: Atrial (Regular) Irregular Ventricular (Regular) Irregular

P WAVES: Upright PR: 0.16s QRS: 0.12s QT: 0.36s Consider QT$_c$ (rate)

ST SEGMENT: (Okay) Elevated Depressed T WAVES: Upright

7.

Sinus tachycardia w/ ST depression

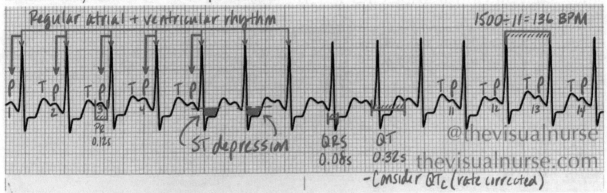

(6 second method)   (Small box method)

RATE: Atrial: 140   Ventricular: 140   Ventricular: 136

RHYTHM: Atrial (Regular) Irregular   Ventricular (Regular) Irregular

P WAVES: Upright PR: 0.12s   QRS: 0.08s   QT: 0.32s Consider QT$_c$ (rate)

ST SEGMENT: Okay Elevated (Depressed)   T WAVES: Upright

8.

Atrial fibrillation with an uncontrolled ventricular response

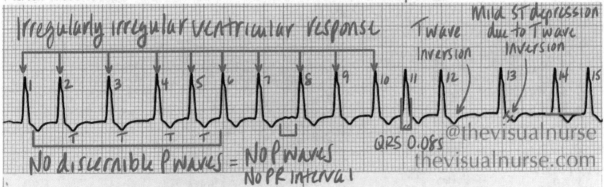

(6 second method)   6 second method preferred for irregular rhythms

(Small box method)

RATE: ~~Atrial:~~ N/A   Ventricular: 150   ~~Ventricular:~~

RHYTHM: ~~Atrial Regular Irregular~~   Ventricular Regular (Irregular)

P WAVES: N/A PR: N/A   QRS: 0.08s   QT: N/A or UTD

ST SEGMENT: Okay Elevated (Depressed)   T WAVES: Inverted

UTD: Unable to determine

9.

Sinus bradycardia with wide QRS and ST depression

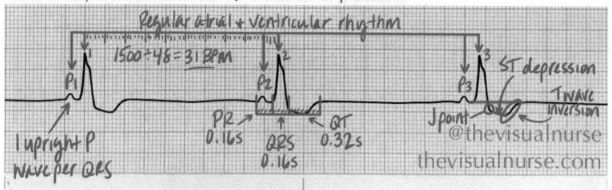

(6 second method)   (Small box method)

RATE: Atrial: __30__ Ventricular: __30__   Ventricular: __31__

RHYTHM: Atrial (Regular) Irregular   Ventricular (Regular) Irregular

P WAVES: Upright PR: 0.16s QRS: 0.16s QT: 0.32s

ST SEGMENT: Okay Elevated (Depressed)   T WAVES: Inverted

10.

Sinus bradycardia with ST depression

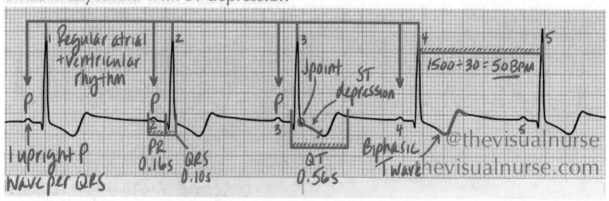

(6 second method)   (Small box method)

RATE: Atrial: __50__ Ventricular: __50__   Ventricular: __50__

RHYTHM: Atrial (Regular) Irregular   Ventricular (Regular) Irregular

P WAVES: Upright PR: 0.16s QRS: 0.10s QT: 0.56s

ST SEGMENT: Okay Elevated (Depressed)   T WAVES: Biphasic

11.

Sinus rhythm with a wide QRS and ST depression

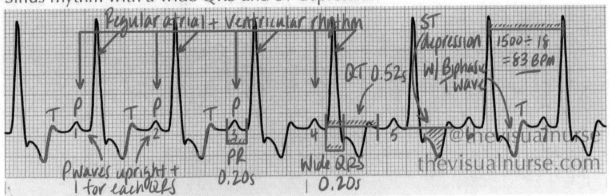

(6 second method)   (Small box method)

RATE: Atrial: _70_ Ventricular: _80_ Ventricular: _83_

RHYTHM: Atrial (Regular) Irregular Ventricular (Regular) Irregular

P WAVES: Upright PR: 0.20s QRS: 0.20s QT: 0.52s

ST SEGMENT: Okay Elevated (Depressed) T WAVES: Biphasic

12.

Sinus rhythm with rate variation (Sinus arrhythmia)

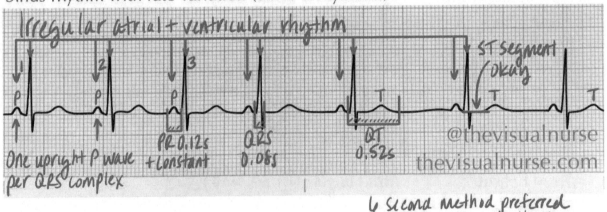

6 second method preferred
for irregular rhythms

(6 second method)   (Small box method)

RATE: Atrial: _70_ Ventricular: _70_ Ventricular: _____

RHYTHM: Atrial Regular (Irregular) Ventricular Regular (Irregular)

P WAVES: upright PR: 0.12s QRS: 0.08s QT: 0.52s

ST SEGMENT: (Okay) Elevated Depressed T WAVES: upright

13.

Atrial tachycardia

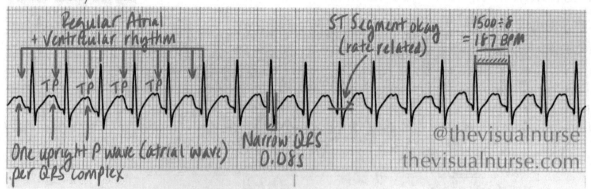

(6 second method)   (Small box method)
RATE: Atrial: 170   Ventricular: 170   Ventricular: 187
RHYTHM: Atrial (Regular) Irregular   Ventricular (Regular) Irregular
P WAVES: Upright PR: UTD QRS: 0.08s QT: UTD
ST SEGMENT: (Okay) Elevated Depressed   T WAVES: Upright
UTD: Unable to determine

14.

Ectopic atrial rhythm

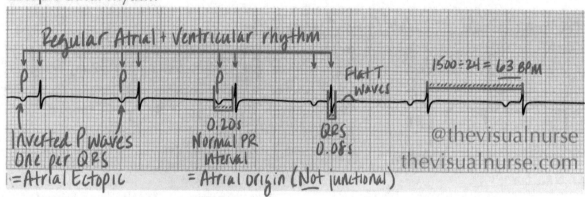

(6 second method)   (Small box method)
RATE: Atrial: 60   Ventricular: 60   Ventricular: 63
RHYTHM: Atrial (Regular) Irregular   Ventricular (Regular) Irregular
P WAVES: Inverted PR: 0.20s QRS: 0.08s QT: UTD
ST SEGMENT: (Okay) Elevated Depressed   T WAVES: Flat
UTD: Unable to determine

15.

Sinus rhythm with ST depression and premature atrial contractions

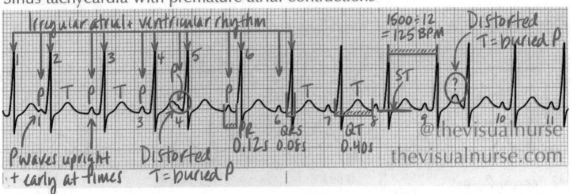

(6 second method)

RATE: Atrial: __60__   Ventricular: __60__   ~~Ventricular:~~ _____

RHYTHM: <u>Atrial</u> Regular (Irregular)   <u>Ventricular</u> Regular (Irregular)

P WAVES: <u>Upright</u> PR: <u>Varies</u>   QRS: <u>0.12s</u> QT: <u>0.52s</u>

ST SEGMENT: Okay Elevated (Depressed)   T WAVES: <u>Biphasic</u>

6 second method preferred for irregular rhythms
~~(Small box method)~~

16.

Sinus tachycardia with premature atrial contractions

(6 second method)   (Small box method)

RATE: Atrial: __110__ Ventricular: __130__   Ventricular: __125__ *

RHYTHM: <u>Atrial</u> Regular (Irregular)   <u>Ventricular</u> Regular (Irregular)

P WAVES: <u>Upright</u> PR: <u>0.12s</u> QRS: <u>0.08s</u> QT: <u>0.40s</u>

ST SEGMENT: (Okay) Elevated Depressed   T WAVES: <u>Upright</u>

* Underlying rhythm, excluding early beats

17.

Sinus rhythm/ sinus tachycardia with premature atrial contractions

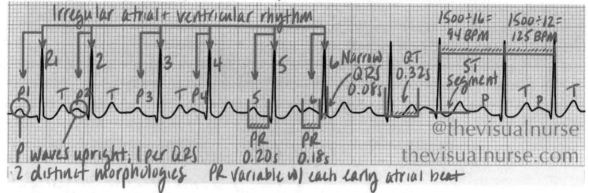

(6 second method)

RATE: Atrial: 100   Ventricular: 100

(Small box method)

Ventricular: 94-125 *

RHYTHM: Atrial Regular (Irregular)   Ventricular Regular (Irregular)

P WAVES: Upright PR: Variable QRS: 0.08s QT: 0.32s

ST SEGMENT: (Okay) Elevated Depressed   T WAVES: Upright

* 6 second method recommended

18.

Sinus rhythm with rate variation (Sinus arrhythmia)

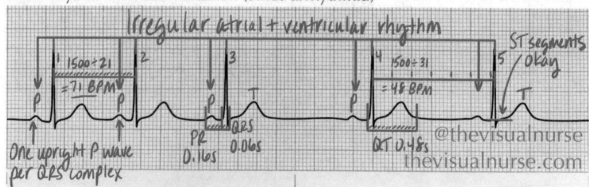

6 second method preferred
for irregular rhythms

(6 second method)

RATE: Atrial: 50   Ventricular: 50

(Small box method)

Ventricular: 48-71 *

RHYTHM: Atrial Regular (Irregular)   Ventricular Regular (Irregular)

P WAVES: Upright PR: 0.16s QRS: 0.06s QT: 0.48s

ST SEGMENT: (Okay) Elevated Depressed   T WAVES: Upright

* In this example we can see why the 6 second method is preferred for rapid approximation

19.

Sinus rhythm with premature atrial contractions

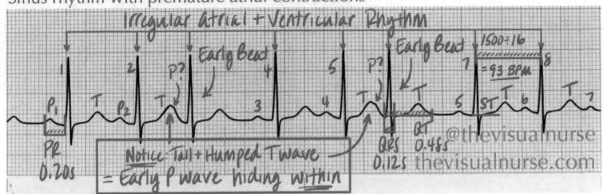

(6 second method)   (Small box method)

RATE: Atrial: _70_* Ventricular: _80_   Ventricular: _93_*

RHYTHM: <u>Atrial</u> Regular (Irregular) <u>Ventricular</u> Regular (Irregular)

P WAVES: <u>Upright</u> PR: _0.20s_ QRS: _0.12s_ QT: _0.48s_

ST SEGMENT: (Okay) Elevated Depressed   T WAVES: Upright

* Underlying rhythm, excluding early beats

20.

Wandering atrial pacemaker

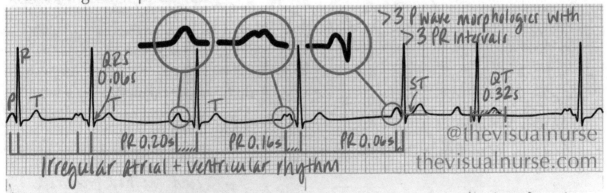

6 second method preferred for irregular rhythms
~~(Small box method)~~

(6 second method)

RATE: Atrial: _70_ Ventricular: _70_   ~~Ventricular:~~

RHYTHM: <u>Atrial</u> Regular (Irregular) <u>Ventricular</u> Regular (Irregular)

P WAVES: <u>Variable</u> PR: <u>Variable</u> QRS: _0.06s_ QT: _0.32s_

ST SEGMENT: (Okay) Elevated Depressed   T WAVES: Upright

21.

Atrial fibrillation with an uncontrolled ventricular response

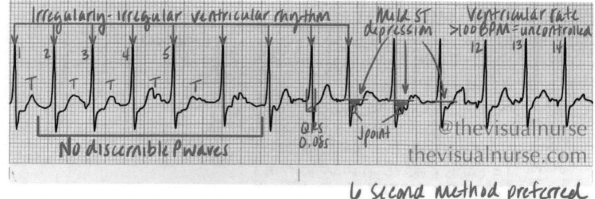

6 second method preferred
for irregular rhythms
(Small box method)

(6 second method)

RATE: ~~Atrial:~~ N/A   Ventricular: 140   ~~Ventricular:~~ _____

RHYTHM: ~~Atrial Regular Irregular~~   Ventricular Regular (Irregular)

P WAVES: N/A   PR: N/A   QRS: 0.08s   QT: N/A or UTD

ST SEGMENT: Okay Elevated (Depressed)   T WAVES: Upright

UTD - Unable to determine

22.

Multifocal atrial tachycardia

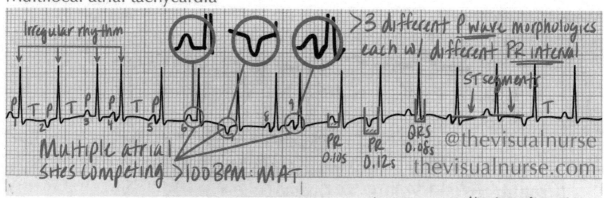

6 second method preferred
for irregular rhythms
(Small box method)

(6 second method)

RATE: Atrial: 160   Ventricular: 160   ~~Ventricular:~~ _____

RHYTHM: Atrial Regular (Irregular)   Ventricular Regular (Irregular)

P WAVES: Variable PR: Variable QRS: 0.08s QT: UTD

ST SEGMENT: (Okay) Elevated Depressed   T WAVES: Flat

UTD: Unable to determine

23.

Atrial fibrillation with an uncontrolled ventricular response

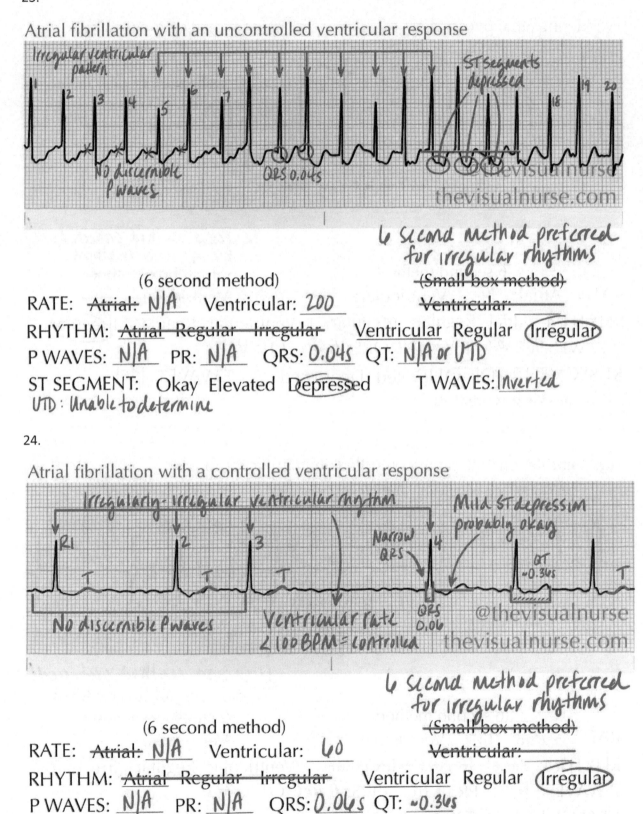

6 second method preferred for irregular rhythms

(6 second method) ~~(Small box method)~~

RATE: ~~Atrial:~~ N/A   Ventricular: 200   ~~Ventricular:~~

RHYTHM: ~~Atrial Regular Irregular~~   Ventricular Regular (Irregular)

P WAVES: N/A   PR: N/A   QRS: 0.04s   QT: N/A or UTD

ST SEGMENT: Okay Elevated (Depressed)   T WAVES: Inverted

UTD: Unable to determine

24.

Atrial fibrillation with a controlled ventricular response

6 second method preferred for irregular rhythms

(6 second method) ~~(Small box method)~~

RATE: ~~Atrial:~~ N/A   Ventricular: 60   ~~Ventricular:~~

RHYTHM: ~~Atrial Regular Irregular~~   Ventricular Regular (Irregular)

P WAVES: N/A   PR: N/A   QRS: 0.06s   QT: ~0.36s

ST SEGMENT: Okay Elevated (Depressed)   T WAVES: Upright/Biphasic

25.

Wandering atrial pacemaker

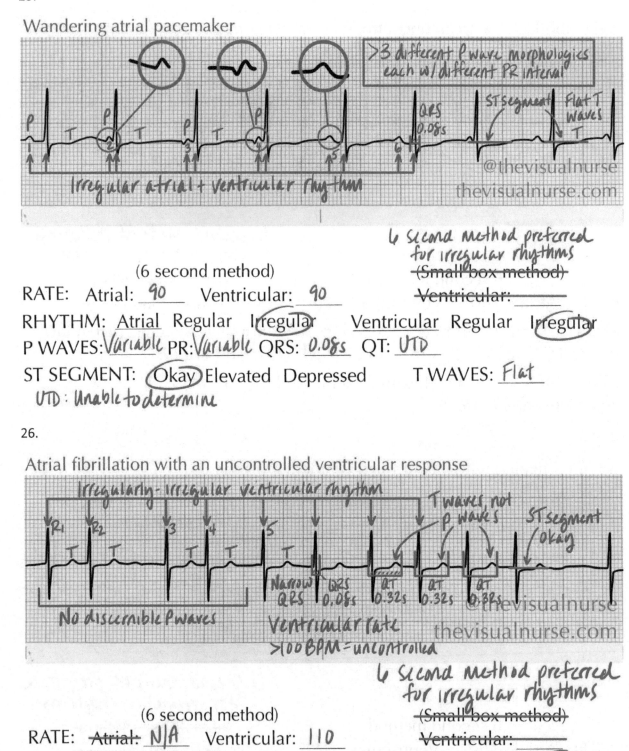

>3 different P wave morphologies each w/ different PR interval

QRS 0.08s

ST segment

Flat T waves T

@thevisualnurse
thevisualnurse.com

Irregular atrial + ventricular rhythm

(6 second method)

6 second method preferred for irregular rhythms
~~(Small box method)~~

RATE: Atrial: 90   Ventricular: 90   ~~Ventricular:~~

RHYTHM: <u>Atrial</u> Regular (Irregular)   <u>Ventricular</u> Regular (Irregular)

P WAVES: Variable PR: Variable QRS: 0.08s QT: UTD

ST SEGMENT: (Okay) Elevated Depressed   T WAVES: Flat

UTD: Unable to determine

26.

Atrial fibrillation with an uncontrolled ventricular response

Irregularly-irregular ventricular rhythm

R1 R2 3 4 5

T waves not P waves

ST segment Okay

Narrow QRS 0.08s QT 0.32s QT 0.32s QT 0.32s

@thevisualnurse
thevisualnurse.com

No discernible P waves

Ventricular rate >100 BPM = uncontrolled

6 second method preferred for irregular rhythms
~~(Small box method)~~

(6 second method)

RATE: ~~Atrial:~~ N/A Ventricular: 110   ~~Ventricular:~~

RHYTHM: ~~Atrial Regular Irregular~~   <u>Ventricular</u> Regular (Irregular)

P WAVES: N/A PR: N/A QRS: 0.08s QT: 0.32s

ST SEGMENT: (Okay) Elevated Depressed   T WAVES: Upright

27.

Atrial fibrillation with an uncontrolled ventricular response

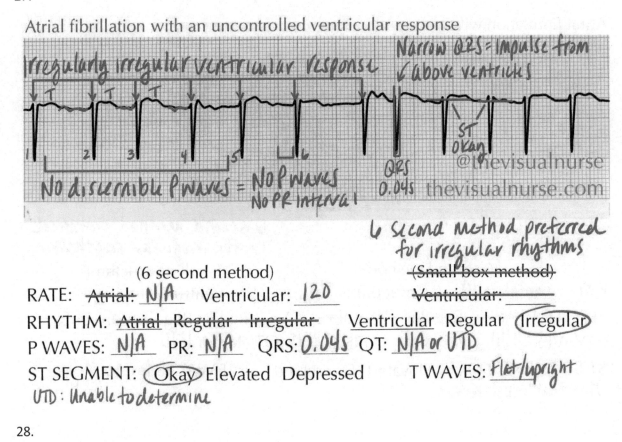

(6 second method)

RATE: ~~Atrial:~~ N/A   Ventricular: 120   ~~Ventricular:~~ _____

(Small box method)

6 second method preferred for irregular rhythms

RHYTHM: ~~Atrial Regular Irregular~~   Ventricular Regular (Irregular)

P WAVES: N/A   PR: N/A   QRS: 0.04s   QT: N/A or UTD

ST SEGMENT: (Okay) Elevated Depressed   T WAVES: Flat/upright

UTD: Unable to determine

28.

Accelerated junctional rhythm

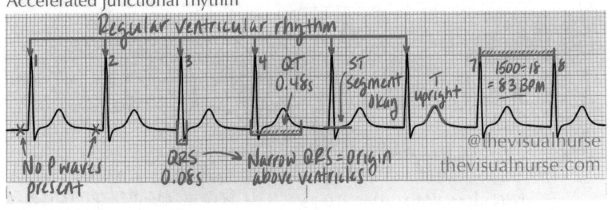

(6 second method)   (Small box method)

RATE: Atrial: N/A   Ventricular: 80   Ventricular: 83

RHYTHM: ~~Atrial Regular Irregular~~   Ventricular (Regular) Irregular

P WAVES: N/A   PR: N/A   QRS: 0.08s   QT: 0.48s

ST SEGMENT: (Okay) Elevated Depressed   T WAVES: Upright

29.

Atrial fibrillation with a controlled ventricular response

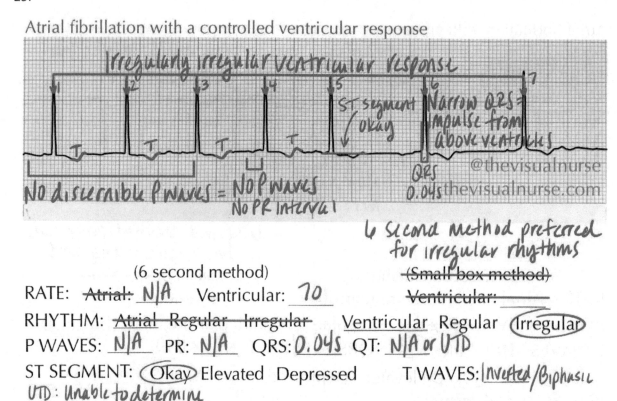

(6 second method)

RATE: ~~Atrial:~~ N/A   Ventricular: 70   ~~Ventricular:~~

RHYTHM: ~~Atrial~~ ~~Regular~~ ~~Irregular~~   Ventricular Regular (Irregular)

P WAVES: N/A   PR: N/A   QRS: 0.04s   QT: N/A or UTD

ST SEGMENT: (Okay) Elevated Depressed   T WAVES: Inverted / Biphasic

UTD: Unable to determine

30.

Atrial fibrillation with a controlled ventricular response

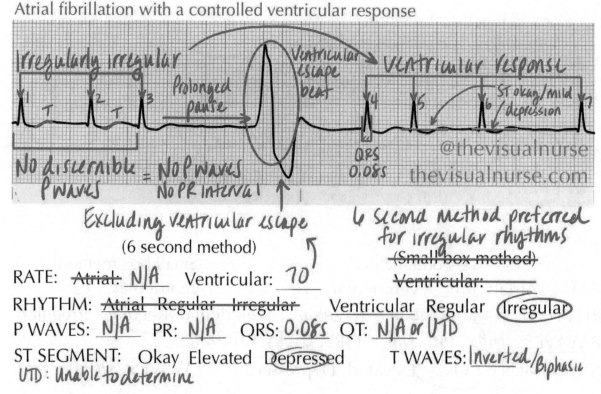

Excluding ventricular escape

(6 second method)

RATE: ~~Atrial:~~ N/A   Ventricular: 70   ~~Ventricular:~~

RHYTHM: ~~Atrial~~ ~~Regular~~ ~~Irregular~~   Ventricular Regular (Irregular)

P WAVES: N/A   PR: N/A   QRS: 0.08s   QT: N/A or UTD

ST SEGMENT: Okay Elevated (Depressed)   T WAVES: Inverted / Biphasic

UTD: Unable to determine

31.

Atrial fibrillation with a controlled ventricular response and T wave inversion

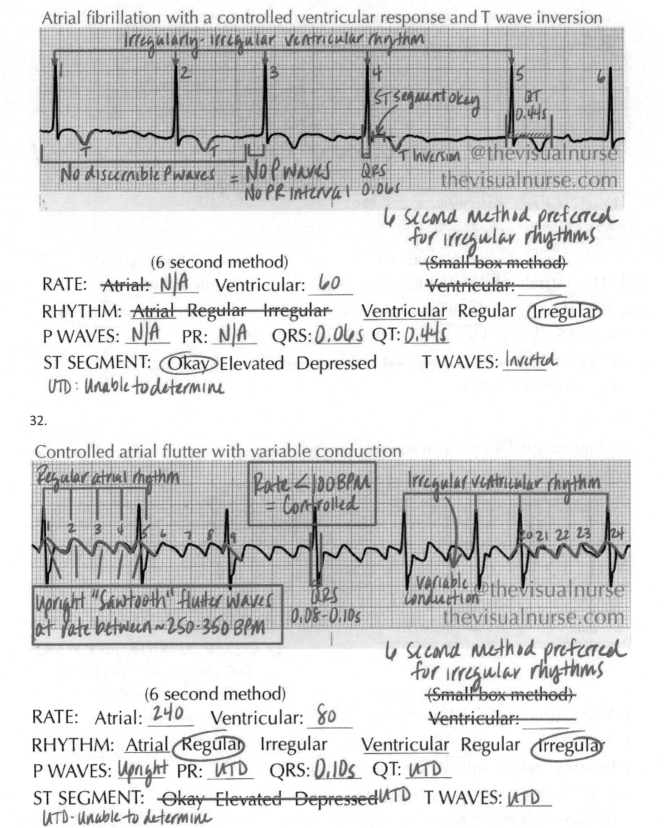

(6 second method)   (Small box method)

RATE: ~~Atrial:~~ N/A   Ventricular: 60   ~~Ventricular:~~

RHYTHM: ~~Atrial Regular Irregular~~ Ventricular Regular (Irregular)

P WAVES: N/A PR: N/A QRS: 0.06s QT: 0.44s

ST SEGMENT: (Okay) Elevated Depressed   T WAVES: Inverted

UTD: Unable to determine

32.

Controlled atrial flutter with variable conduction

(6 second method)   (Small box method)

RATE: Atrial: 240 Ventricular: 80   ~~Ventricular:~~

RHYTHM: Atrial (Regular) Irregular Ventricular Regular (Irregular)

P WAVES: Upright PR: UTD QRS: 0.10s QT: UTD

ST SEGMENT: ~~Okay Elevated Depressed~~ UTD T WAVES: UTD

UTD- Unable to determine

33.

Atrial flutter with 3:1 conduction

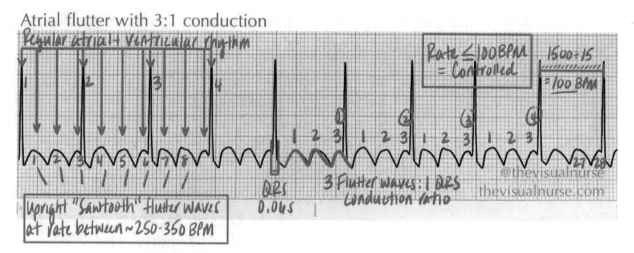

RATE: Atrial: <u>280</u>   Ventricular: <u>100</u>   (6 second method)   Ventricular: <u>100</u>   (Small box method)

RHYTHM: Atrial <u>Regular</u> (Regular) Irregular   Ventricular <u>Regular</u> (Irregular)

P WAVES: <u>Upright</u>   PR: <u>UTD</u>   QRS: <u>0.04s</u>   QT: <u>UTD</u>

ST SEGMENT: ~~Okay Elevated Depressed~~ UTD   **T WAVES:** <u>UTD</u>

UTD - Unable to determine

34.

Controlled atrial flutter with variable conduction

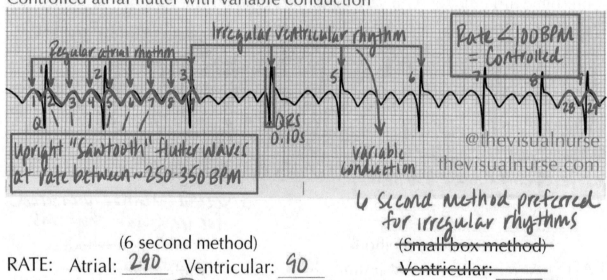

6 second method preferred for irregular rhythms

RATE: Atrial: <u>290</u>   Ventricular: <u>90</u>   (6 second method)   ~~(Small box method)~~   ~~Ventricular:~~

RHYTHM: Atrial <u>Regular</u> (Regular) Irregular   Ventricular <u>Regular</u> (Irregular)

P WAVES: <u>Upright</u>   PR: <u>UTD</u>   QRS: <u>0.10s</u>   QT: <u>UTD</u>

ST SEGMENT: ~~Okay Elevated Depressed~~ UTD   **T WAVES:** <u>UTD</u>

UTD - Unable to determine

35.

Junctional rhythm with flat T waves

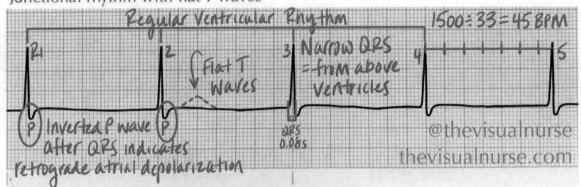

(6 second method) | (Small box method)

RATE: Atrial: N/A* Ventricular: 50 | Ventricular: 45

RHYTHM: ~~Atrial Regular Irregular~~* Ventricular (Regular) Irregular

P WAVES: Inverted PR: N/A* QRS: 0.08s QT: UTD

ST SEGMENT: (Okay) Elevated Depressed   T WAVES: Flat

*As measured by intrinsic P waves   UTD= Unable to determine

36.

Idioventricular rhythm

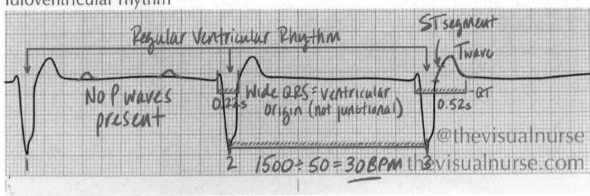

(6 second method) | (Small box method)

RATE: Atrial: N/A Ventricular: 30 | Ventricular: 30

RHYTHM: ~~Atrial Regular Irregular~~ Ventricular (Regular) Irregular

P WAVES: N/A PR: N/A QRS: 0.22s QT: 0.52s

ST SEGMENT: Okay (Elevated) Depressed   T WAVES: Upright

37.

Junctional rhythm

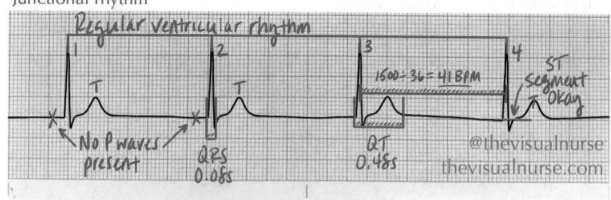

(6 second method) (Small box method)

RATE: Atrial: N/A Ventricular: 40 Ventricular: 41

RHYTHM: ~~Atrial~~ ~~Regular~~ ~~Irregular~~ Ventricular (Regular) Irregular

P WAVES: N/A PR: N/A QRS: 0.08s QT: 0.48s

ST SEGMENT: (Okay) Elevated Depressed T WAVES: Upright

38.

Sinus tachycardia with premature junctional contractions

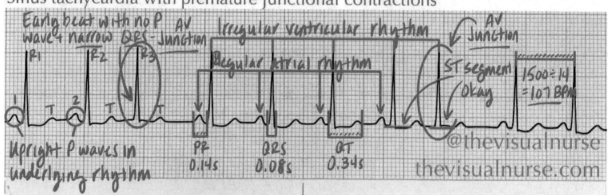

(6 second method) (Small box method)

RATE: Atrial: 80 Ventricular: 100 Ventricular: 107

RHYTHM: Atrial (Regular)* Irregular Ventricular Regular (Irregular)

P WAVES: Upright PR: 0.14s QRS: 0.08s QT: 0.34s

ST SEGMENT: (Okay) Elevated Depressed T WAVES: Upright

*For the underlying rhythm

39.

Accelerated junctional rhythm

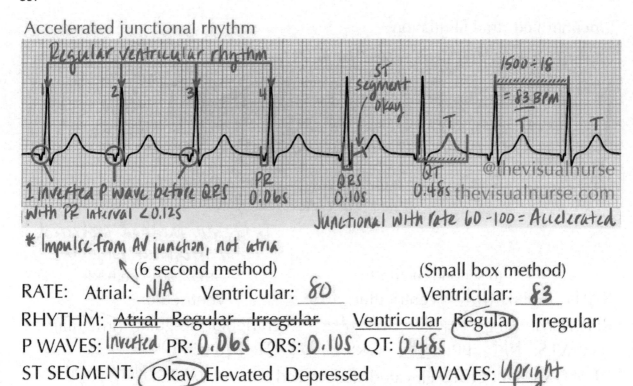

* Impulse from AV junction, not atria

↖ (6 second method)   (Small box method)

RATE: Atrial: __NIA__ Ventricular: __80__   Ventricular: __83__

RHYTHM: ~~Atrial Regular Irregular~~   Ventricular (Regular) Irregular

P WAVES: __Inverted__ PR: __0.06s__ QRS: __0.10s__ QT: __0.48s__

ST SEGMENT: (Okay) Elevated Depressed   T WAVES: __Upright__

40.

Junctional tachycardia with ST depression

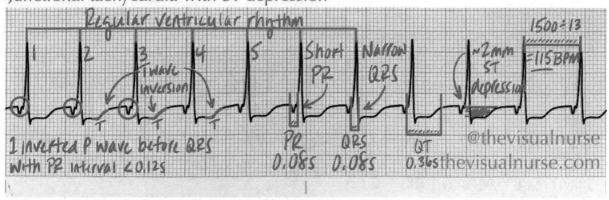

* Impulse from AV junction, not atria

↖ (6 second method)   (Small box method)

RATE: Atrial: __NIA__ Ventricular: __110__   Ventricular: __115__

RHYTHM: ~~Atrial Regular Irregular~~   Ventricular (Regular) Irregular

P WAVES: __Inverted__ PR: __0.08s__ QRS: __0.08s__ QT: __0.36s__

ST SEGMENT: Okay Elevated (Depressed)   T WAVES: __Inverted__

41.

Uncontrolled atrial fibrillation

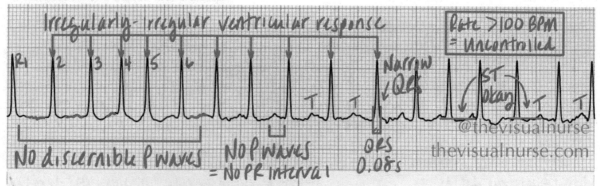

(6 second method)

RATE: ~~Atrial:~~ N/A   Ventricular: 170   ~~(Small box method)~~ ~~Ventricular:~~_____

RHYTHM: ~~Atrial Regular Irregular~~   Ventricular Regular (Irregular)

P WAVES: N/A   PR: N/A   QRS: 0.08s   QT: N/A or UTD

ST SEGMENT: (Okay) Elevated Depressed   T WAVES: Flat/upright

UTD: Unable to determine

42.

Junctional tachycardia with flat T waves

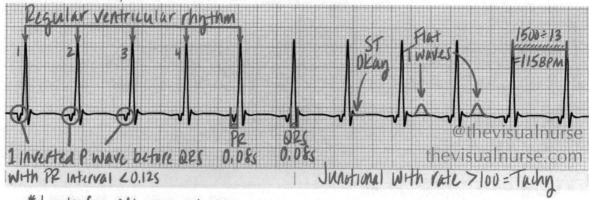

* Impulse from AV junction, not atria

(6 second method)   (Small box method)

RATE: Atrial: N/A   Ventricular: 110   Ventricular: 115

RHYTHM: ~~Atrial Regular Irregular~~   Ventricular (Regular) Irregular

P WAVES: Inverted PR: 0.08s QRS: 0.08s QT: UTD

ST SEGMENT: (Okay) Elevated Depressed   T WAVES: Flat

UTD - Unable to determine

43.

Supraventricular tachycardia with ST depression

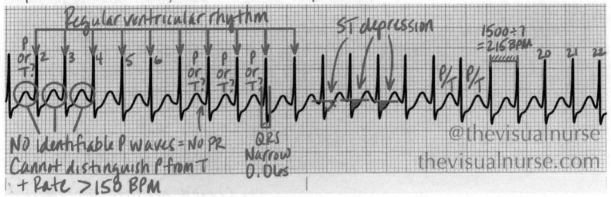

*No discernible P waves
↖ (6 second method)   (Small box method)

RATE: Atrial: N/A   Ventricular: 220   Ventricular: 215

RHYTHM: ~~Atrial Regular Irregular~~   Ventricular (Regular) Irregular

P WAVES: N/A   PR: N/A   QRS: 0.06s   QT: N/A or UTD

ST SEGMENT: Okay   Elevated   (Depressed)   T WAVES: N/A or upright

UTD - Unable to determine

44.

Supraventricular tachycardia with ST depression

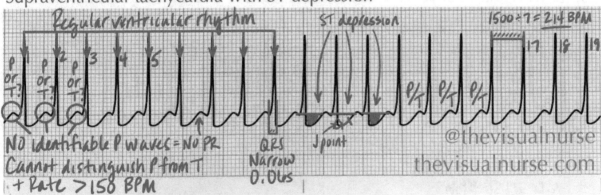

*No discernible P waves
↖ (6 second method)   (Small box method)

RATE: Atrial: N/A   Ventricular: 190   Ventricular: 214

RHYTHM: ~~Atrial Regular Irregular~~   Ventricular (Regular) Irregular

P WAVES: N/A   PR: N/A   QRS: 0.06s   QT: N/A or UTD

ST SEGMENT: Okay   Elevated   (Depressed)   T WAVES: N/A or upright

UTD - Unable to determine

45.

Atrial fibrillation with an uncontrolled ventricular response and ST depression

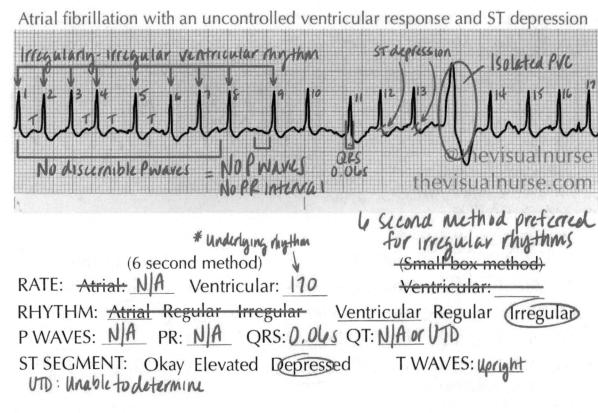

* Underlying rhythm

(6 second method)

6 second method preferred for irregular rhythms
~~(Small box method)~~

RATE: ~~Atrial:~~ N/A   Ventricular: 170   ~~Ventricular:~~ _____

RHYTHM: ~~Atrial Regular Irregular~~   Ventricular Regular (Irregular)

P WAVES: N/A   PR: N/A   QRS: 0.06s   QT: N/A or UTD

ST SEGMENT: Okay Elevated (Depressed)   T WAVES: Upright

UTD: Unable to determine

46.

Supraventricular tachycardia with ST depression

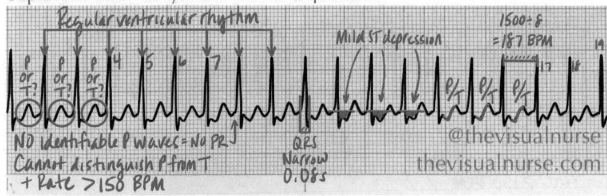

* No discernible P waves

(6 second method)   (Small box method)

RATE: Atrial: N/A   Ventricular: 190   Ventricular: 187

RHYTHM: ~~Atrial Regular Irregular~~   Ventricular (Regular) Irregular

P WAVES: N/A   PR: N/A   QRS: 0.08s   QT: N/A or UTD

ST SEGMENT: Okay Elevated (Depressed)   T WAVES: N/A or Biphasic

UTD - Unable to determine

47.

Sinus tachycardia with ST depression

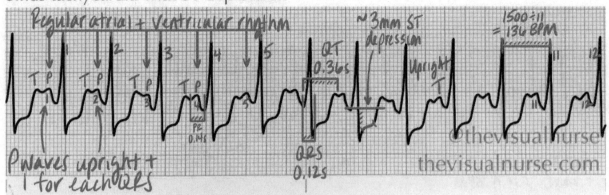

(6 second method)   (Small box method)

RATE: Atrial: 120   Ventricular: 120   Ventricular: 136

RHYTHM: Atrial (Regular) Irregular   Ventricular (Regular) Irregular

P WAVES: Upright   PR: 0.14s   QRS: 0.12s   QT: 0.36s Consider QTc (rate)

ST SEGMENT: Okay Elevated (Depressed)   T WAVES: Upright

48.

Supraventricular tachycardia with ST depression

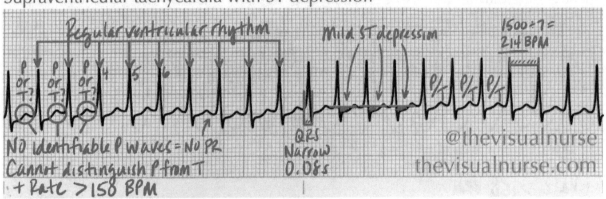

*No discernible P waves

(6 second method)   (Small box method)

RATE: Atrial: N/A   Ventricular: 210   Ventricular: 214

RHYTHM: ~~Atrial Regular Irregular~~   Ventricular (Regular) Irregular

P WAVES: N/A   PR: N/A   QRS: 0.08s   QT: N/A or UTD

ST SEGMENT: Okay Elevated (Depressed)   T WAVES: N/A or upright

UTD - Unable to determine

49.

Supraventricular tachycardia with ST depression

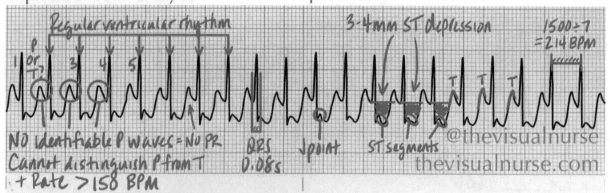

*No discernible P waves
↖ (6 second method)   (Small box method)

RATE: Atrial: N/A   200   Ventricular: 214

RHYTHM: ~~Atrial~~ ~~Regular~~ ~~Irregular~~   Ventricular (Regular) Irregular

P WAVES: N/A   PR: N/A   QRS: 0.08s QT: N/A or UTD

ST SEGMENT: Okay Elevated (Depressed)   T WAVES: Upright/Biphasic
UTD - Unable to determine

50.

Supraventricular tachycardia with ST depression

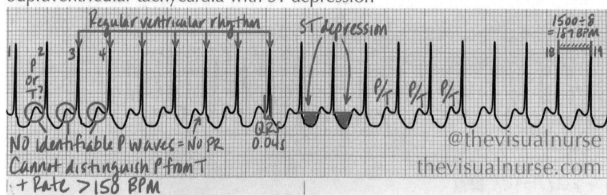

*No discernible P waves
↖ (6 second method)   (Small box method)

RATE: Atrial: N/A   Ventricular: 190   Ventricular: 187

RHYTHM: ~~Atrial~~ ~~Regular~~ ~~Irregular~~   Ventricular (Regular) Irregular

P WAVES: N/A   PR: N/A   QRS: 0.04s QT: N/A or UTD

ST SEGMENT: Okay Elevated (Depressed)   T WAVES: N/A or upright
UTD - Unable to determine

51.

Sinus bradycardia with a first degree AV delay, ventricular bigeminy and downsloping ST depression

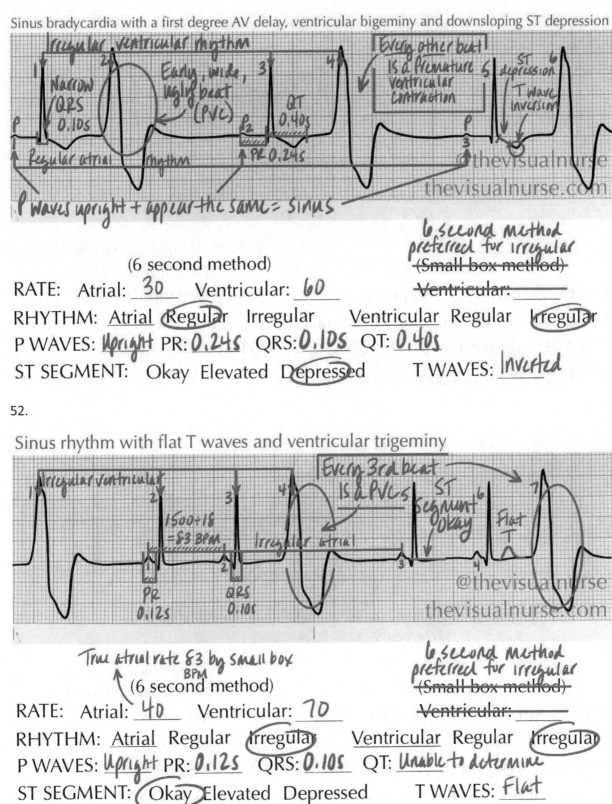

(6 second method)

RATE: Atrial: 30   Ventricular: 60   Ventricular: ~~~~

RHYTHM: Atrial (Regular) Irregular   Ventricular Regular (Irregular)

P WAVES: Upright PR: 0.24s QRS: 0.10s QT: 0.40s

ST SEGMENT: Okay Elevated (Depressed)   T WAVES: Inverted

52.

Sinus rhythm with flat T waves and ventricular trigeminy

True atrial rate 83 by small box BPM

(6 second method)

RATE: Atrial: 40   Ventricular: 70   Ventricular: ~~~~

RHYTHM: Atrial Regular (Irregular)   Ventricular Regular (Irregular)

P WAVES: Upright PR: 0.12s QRS: 0.10s QT: Unable to determine

ST SEGMENT: (Okay) Elevated Depressed   T WAVES: Flat

53.

Sinus rhythm with a multifocal ventricular couplet

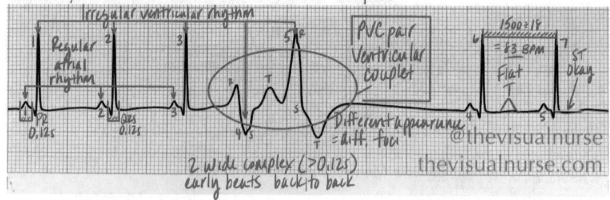

(6 second method)

Underlying rhythm
(Small box method)

RATE: Atrial: __50__ Ventricular: __70__   Ventricular: __83__

RHYTHM: Atrial (Regular) Irregular   Ventricular Regular (Irregular)

P WAVES: Upright PR: __0.12s__ QRS: __0.12s__ QT: Unable to determine

ST SEGMENT: (Okay) Elevated Depressed   T WAVES: Flat

54.

Sinus rhythm with a ventricular couplet

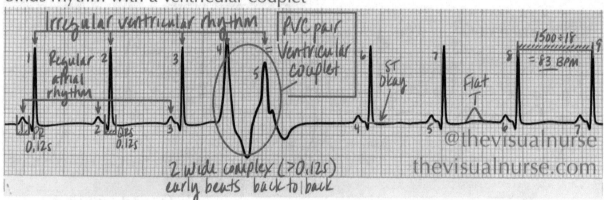

(6 second method)

Underlying rhythm
(Small box method)

RATE: Atrial: __70__ Ventricular: __90__   Ventricular: __83__

RHYTHM: Atrial (Regular) Irregular   Ventricular Regular (Irregular)

P WAVES: Upright PR: __0.12s__ QRS: __0.12s__ QT: Unable to determine

ST SEGMENT: (Okay) Elevated Depressed

T WAVES: Flat

55.

Idioventricular rhythm

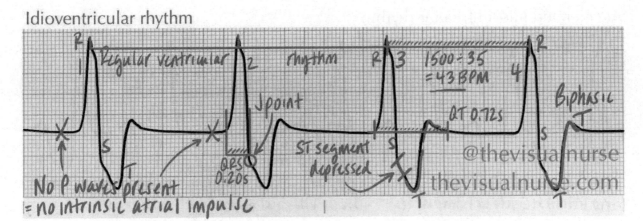

(6 second method)   (Small box method)

RATE: Atrial: __N/A__ Ventricular: __40__   Ventricular: __43__

RHYTHM: ~~Atrial Regular Irregular~~ Ventricular (Regular) Irregular

P WAVES: __N/A__ PR: __N/A__ QRS: __0.20s__ QT: __0.72s__ (likely inaccurate)

ST SEGMENT: Okay Elevated (Depressed)   T WAVES: Biphasic

56.

Accelerated idioventricular rhythm

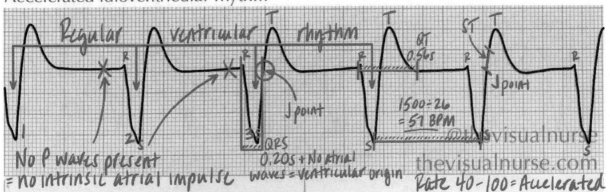

(6 second method)   (Small box method)

RATE: Atrial: __N/A__ Ventricular: __60__   Ventricular: __57__

RHYTHM: ~~Atrial Regular Irregular~~ Ventricular (Regular) Irregular

P WAVES: __N/A__ PR: __N/A__ QRS: __0.20s__ QT: __0.56s__

ST SEGMENT: Okay (Elevated) Depressed   T WAVES: Upright

57.

Accelerated idioventricular rhythm

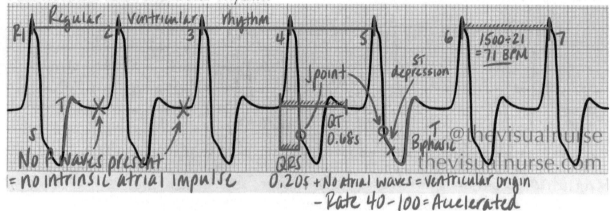

No P waves present
= no intrinsic atrial impulse   0.20s + No atrial waves = ventricular origin
- Rate 40-100 = Accelerated

(6 second method)	(Small box method)

RATE: Atrial: _N/A_   Ventricular: _70_   Ventricular: _71_

RHYTHM: ~~Atrial Regular Irregular~~   Ventricular (Regular) Irregular

P WAVES: _N/A_ PR: _N/A_   QRS: _0.20s_ QT: _0.68s_

ST SEGMENT: Okay Elevated (Depressed)   T WAVES: _Biphasic_

58.

Atrial sensed, ventricular paced rhythm

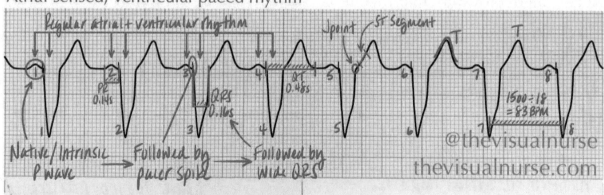

Native/Intrinsic P wave   Followed by pacer spike   Followed by wide QRS

(6 second method)	(Small box method)

RATE: Atrial: _80_   Ventricular: _80_   Ventricular: _83_

RHYTHM: Atrial (Regular) Irregular   Ventricular (Regular) Irregular

P WAVES: _Upright_ PR: _0.14s_   QRS: _0.16s_ QT: _0.48s_

ST SEGMENT: Okay (Elevated) Depressed   T WAVES: _Upright_

59.

Monomorphic ventricular tachycardia

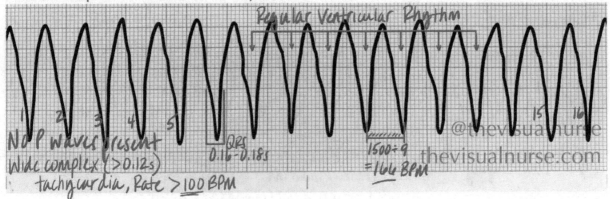

(6 second method)   (Small box method)

RATE: Atrial: N/A   Ventricular: 160   Ventricular: 166

RHYTHM: ~~Atrial Regular Irregular~~   Ventricular (Regular) Irregular

P WAVES: N/A   PR: N/A   QRS: 0.18s   QT: Unable to determine

ST SEGMENT: ~~Okay Elevated Depressed~~   T WAVES: Unable to determine

60.

Monomorphic ventricular tachycardia

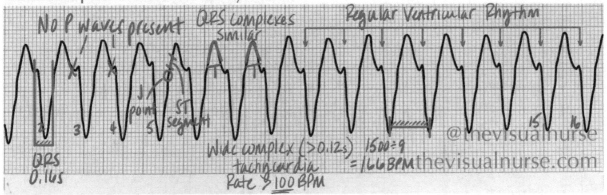

(6 second method)   (Small box method)

RATE: Atrial: N/A   Ventricular: 160   Ventricular: 166

RHYTHM: ~~Atrial Regular Irregular~~   Ventricular (Regular) Irregular

P WAVES: N/A   PR: N/A   QRS: 0.16s   QT: Unable to determine

ST SEGMENT: Okay (Elevated) Depressed   T WAVES: Upright

61.

Sinus rhythm with a run of non-sustained ventricular tachycardia (NSVT)

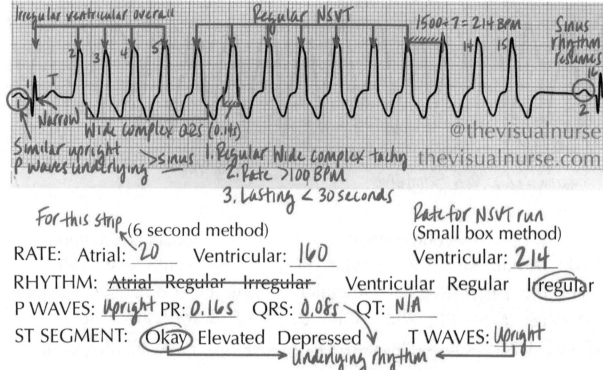

For this strip (6 second method)

RATE: Atrial: 20   Ventricular: 160   Rate for NSVT run (Small box method) Ventricular: 214

RHYTHM: ~~Atrial Regular Irregular~~   Ventricular Regular (Irregular)

P WAVES: Upright PR: 0.16s   QRS: 0.08s QT: N/A

ST SEGMENT: (Okay) Elevated Depressed ↓   T WAVES: Upright
→ Underlying rhythm ←

62.

Polymorphic ventricular tachycardia; Torsades de Pointes

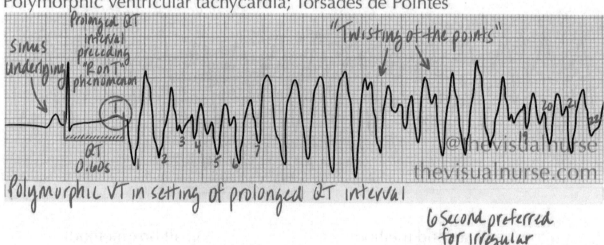

Polymorphic VT in setting of prolonged QT interval

(6 second method)

6 second preferred for irregular

RATE: Atrial: N/A   Ventricular: ~220   ~~(Small box method)~~ ~~Ventricular:~~

RHYTHM: ~~Atrial Regular Irregular~~   Ventricular Regular (Irregular)

P WAVES: N/A PR: N/A   QRS: Wide/variable QT: 0.60s

ST SEGMENT: ~~Okay Elevated Depressed~~   T WAVES: Unable to determine

63.

Sinus/ sinus tachycardia with a run of non-sustained ventricular tachycardia (NSVT)

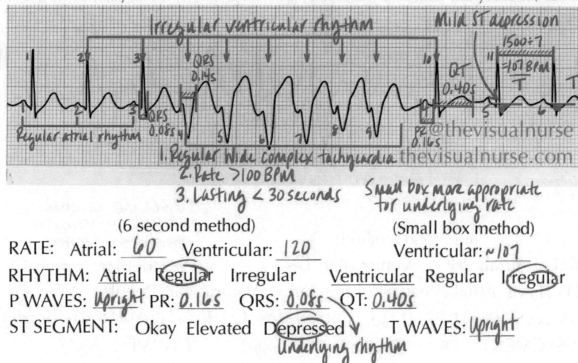

1. Regular Wide complex tachycardia
2. Rate >100 BPM
3. Lasting < 30 seconds

Small box more appropriate for underlying rate

(6 second method)   (Small box method)

RATE: Atrial: 60   Ventricular: 120   Ventricular: ~107

RHYTHM: Atrial Regular Irregular   Ventricular Regular Irregular

P WAVES: Upright PR: 0.16s   QRS: 0.08s   QT: 0.40s

ST SEGMENT: Okay Elevated Depressed ↓   T WAVES: Upright
Underlying rhythm

64.

Non-sustained polymorphic ventricular tachycardia

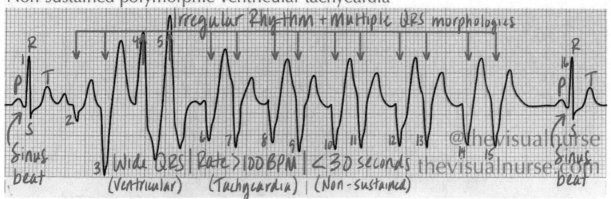

Wide QRS | Rate >100 BPM | < 30 seconds
(Ventricular) | (Tachycardia) | (Non-sustained)

6 second preferred for irregular

(6 second method)   (Small box method)

RATE: Atrial: N/A   Ventricular: 160   Ventricular: _____

RHYTHM: Atrial Regular Irregular   Ventricular Regular Irregular

P WAVES: N/A   PR: N/A   QRS: Wide/Variable   QT: Unable to determine

ST SEGMENT: Okay Elevated Depressed   T WAVES: Unable to determine

65.

Sinus rhythm with ST depression and multifocal PVCs in ventricular bigeminy

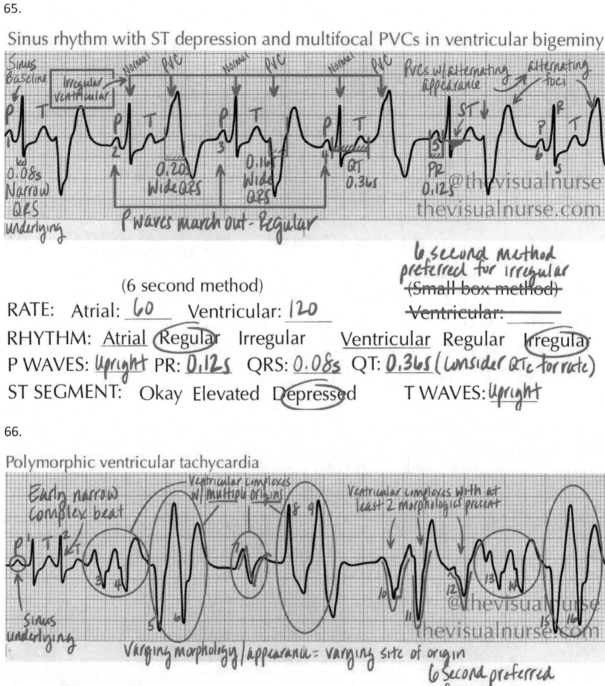

(6 second method)

6 second method preferred for irregular (Small box method)

RATE: Atrial: 60   Ventricular: 120   Ventricular: _____

RHYTHM: Atrial (Regular) Irregular   Ventricular Regular (Irregular)

P WAVES: Upright PR: 0.12s   QRS: 0.08s   QT: 0.36s (Consider QTc for rate)

ST SEGMENT: Okay Elevated (Depressed)   T WAVES: Upright

66.

Polymorphic ventricular tachycardia

Varying morphology / appearance = varying site of origin

(6 second method)

6 second preferred for irregular (Small box method)

RATE: Atrial: N/A   Ventricular: 160   Ventricular: _____

RHYTHM: Atrial Regular Irregular   Ventricular Regular (Irregular)

P WAVES: N/A   PR: N/A   QRS: Wide/Variable   QT: Unable to determine

ST SEGMENT: Okay Elevated Depressed   T WAVES: Unable to determine

67.

Polymorphic ventricular tachycardia; Torsades de Pointes

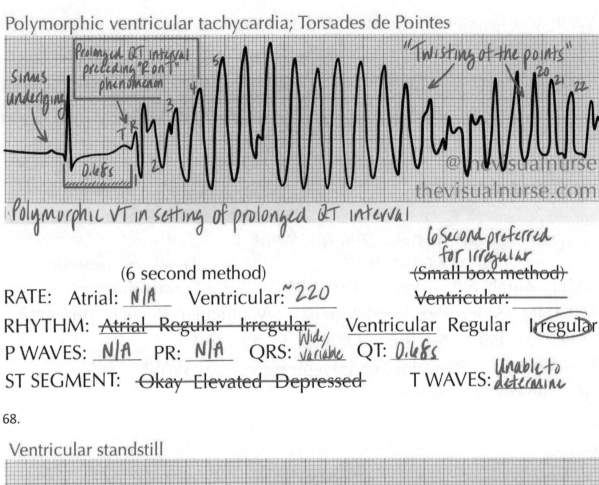

Polymorphic VT in setting of prolonged QT interval

6 second preferred
for irregular

	(6 second method)		~~(Small box method)~~

RATE: Atrial: N/A Ventricular: ~220   ~~Ventricular:~~ _____

RHYTHM: ~~Atrial Regular Irregular~~ Ventricular Regular (Irregular)

P WAVES: N/A PR: N/A QRS: Wide/variable QT: 0.68s

ST SEGMENT: ~~Okay Elevated Depressed~~   T WAVES: Unable to ~~determine~~

68.

Ventricular standstill

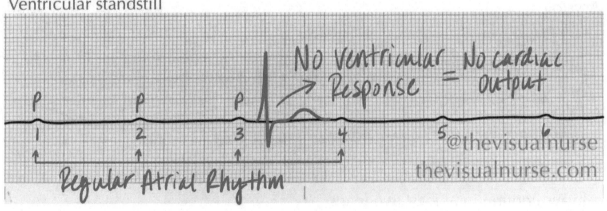

No ventricular Response = No cardiac output

Regular Atrial Rhythm

	(6 second method)		(Small box method)

RATE: Atrial: 60 Ventricular: N/A   Ventricular: N/A

RHYTHM: Atrial (Regular) Irregular ~~Ventricular Regular Irregular~~

P WAVES: Upright PR: N/A QRS: N/A QT: N/A

ST SEGMENT: ~~Okay Elevated Depressed~~   T WAVES: N/A

69.

Ventricular fibrillation

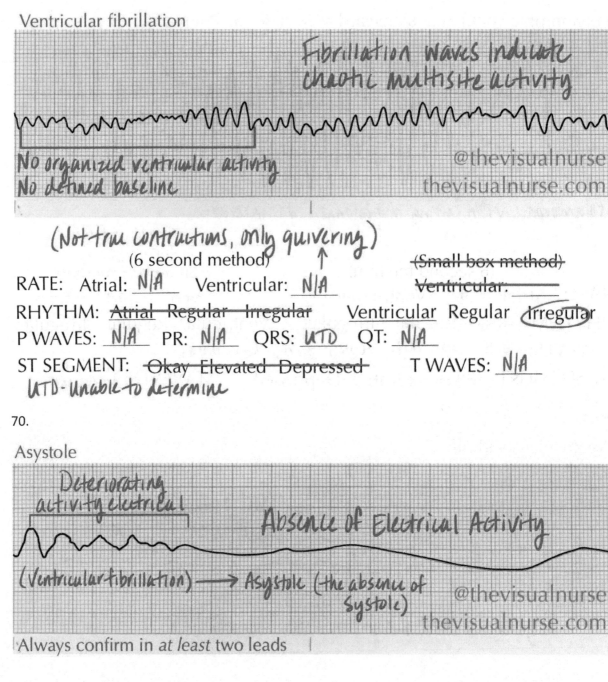

Fibrillation waves indicate chaotic multisite activity

No organized ventricular activity
No defined baseline

@thevisualnurse
thevisualnurse.com

(Not true contractions, only quivering)

(6 second method) ↑   (Small box method)

RATE: Atrial: N/A   Ventricular: N/A   Ventricular: _____

RHYTHM: Atrial Regular Irregular   Ventricular Regular (Irregular)

P WAVES: N/A   PR: N/A   QRS: UTD   QT: N/A

ST SEGMENT: Okay Elevated Depressed   T WAVES: N/A

UTD- Unable to determine

70.

Asystole

Deteriorating
activity electrical

Absence of Electrical Activity

(Ventricular fibrillation) ——→ Asystole (the absence of Systole)

@thevisualnurse
thevisualnurse.com

Always confirm in *at least* two leads

(6 second method)   (Small box method)

RATE: Atrial: N/A   Ventricular: N/A   Ventricular: N/A

RHYTHM: Atrial Regular Irregular   Ventricular Regular Irregular

P WAVES: N/A   PR: N/A   QRS: N/A   QT: N/A

ST SEGMENT: Okay Elevated Depressed   T WAVES: N/A

71.

Asystole

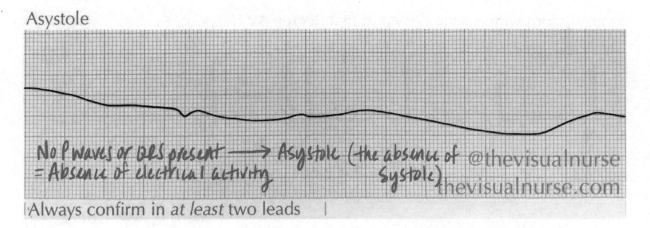

No P waves or QRS present ——→ Asystole (the absence of
= Absence of electrical activity   Systole)

Always confirm in *at least* two leads

(6 second method)   (Small box method)

RATE: Atrial: N/A   Ventricular: N/A   Ventricular: N/A

RHYTHM: ~~Atrial Regular Irregular~~   ~~Ventricular Regular Irregular~~

P WAVES: N/A PR: N/A QRS: N/A QT: N/A

ST SEGMENT: ~~Okay Elevated Depressed~~   T WAVES: N/A

72.

Ventricular fibrillation

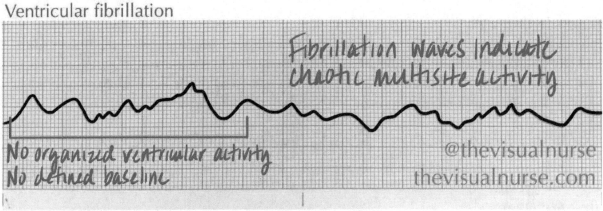

Fibrillation waves indicate
chaotic multisite activity

No organized ventricular activity
No defined baseline

@thevisualnurse
thevisualnurse.com

(Not true contractions, only quivering)

(6 second method)   ↑   ~~(Small box method)~~

RATE: Atrial: N/A   Ventricular: N/A   ~~Ventricular:~~

RHYTHM: ~~Atrial Regular Irregular~~   Ventricular Regular (Irregular)

P WAVES: N/A PR: N/A QRS: UTD QT: N/A

ST SEGMENT: ~~Okay Elevated Depressed~~   T WAVES: N/A

UTD - Unable to determine

73.

Sinus rhythm with a wide QRS and first degree AV delay

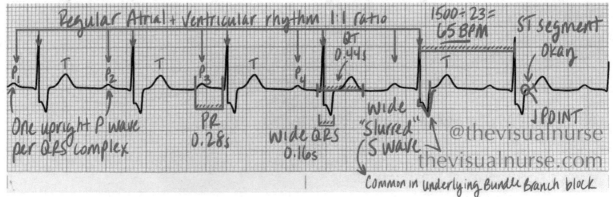

(6 second method)   (Small box method)
RATE: Atrial: 70   Ventricular: 70   Ventricular: 65
RHYTHM: Atrial (Regular) Irregular   Ventricular (Regular) Irregular
P WAVES: Upright PR: 0.28s   QRS: 0.16s QT: 0.44s
ST SEGMENT: (Okay) Elevated Depressed   T WAVES: Upright

74.

Sinus rhythm with a 1st degree AV delay

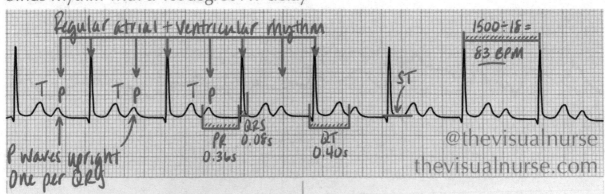

(6 second method)   (Small box method)
RATE: Atrial: 80   Ventricular: 80   Ventricular: 83
RHYTHM: Atrial (Regular) Irregular   Ventricular (Regular) Irregular
P WAVES: upright PR: 0.36s   QRS: 0.08s QT: 0.40s
ST SEGMENT: (Okay) Elevated Depressed   T WAVES: upright

75.

Complete heart block; 3rd degree AV block

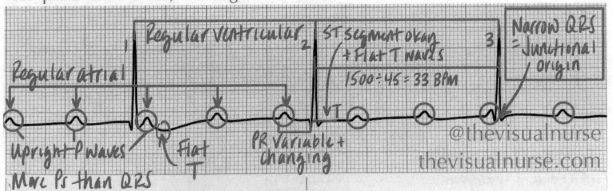

(6 second method)   (Small box method)

RATE: Atrial: __90__ Ventricular: __30__   Ventricular: __33__

RHYTHM: Atrial (Regular) Irregular   Ventricular (Regular) Irregular

P WAVES: Upright PR: Variable QRS: 0.06s QT: Unable to determine

ST SEGMENT: Okay Elevated (Depressed)   T WAVES: Flat

76.

Sinus rhythm/ sinus bradycardia with a 1st degree AV delay

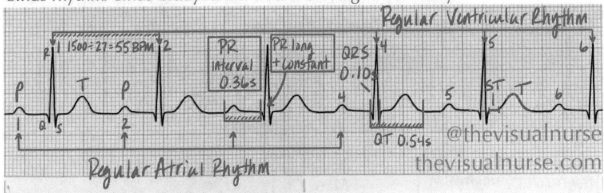

(6 second method)   (Small box method)

RATE: Atrial: __60__ Ventricular: __60__   Ventricular: __55__

RHYTHM: Atrial (Regular) Irregular   Ventricular (Regular) Irregular

P WAVES: upright PR: 0.36s QRS: 0.10s QT: 0.54s

ST SEGMENT: (Okay) Elevated Depressed   T WAVES: upright

77.

Sinus rhythm with second degree type I AV block; Mobitz I; Wenckebach

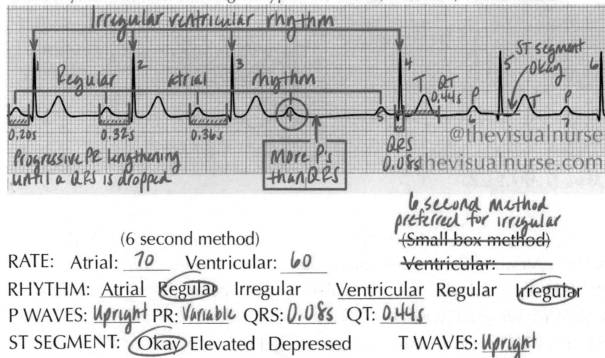

(6 second method)

RATE: Atrial: 70   Ventricular: 60   Ventricular: _____

RHYTHM: Atrial (Regular) Irregular   Ventricular Regular (Irregular)

P WAVES: Upright PR: Variable QRS: 0.08s QT: 0.44s

ST SEGMENT: (Okay) Elevated Depressed   T WAVES: Upright

78.

Sinus rhythm with second degree type I AV block; Mobitz I; Wenckebach

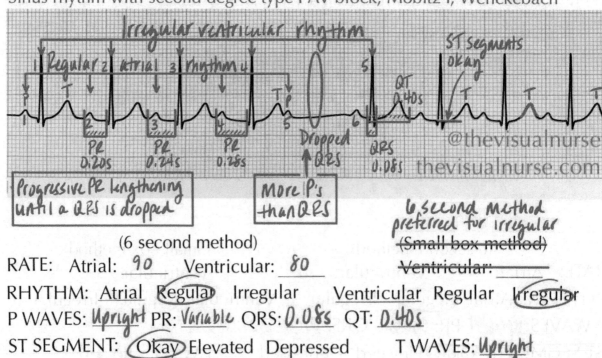

(6 second method)

RATE: Atrial: 90   Ventricular: 80   Ventricular: _____

RHYTHM: Atrial (Regular) Irregular   Ventricular Regular (Irregular)

P WAVES: Upright PR: Variable QRS: 0.08s QT: 0.40s

ST SEGMENT: (Okay) Elevated Depressed   T WAVES: Upright

79.

Sinus rhythm with second degree type I AV block; Mobitz I; Wenckebach

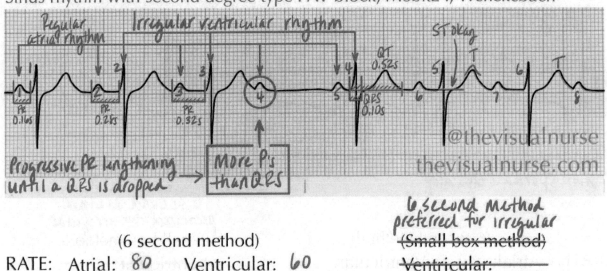

(6 second method)

RATE: Atrial: 80   Ventricular: 60   ~~Ventricular:~~ _____ (Small box method)

RHYTHM: Atrial (Regular) Irregular   Ventricular Regular (Irregular)

P WAVES: Upright PR: Variable QRS: 0.10s QT: 0.52s

ST SEGMENT: (Okay) Elevated Depressed   T WAVES: Upright

80.

Sinus rhythm with second degree type I AV block; Mobitz I; Wenckebach & isolated PVC

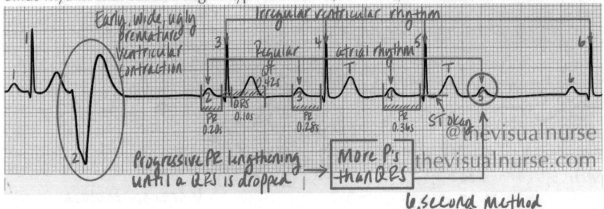

(6 second method)

RATE: Atrial: 60   Ventricular: 60   ~~Ventricular:~~ _____ (Small box method)

RHYTHM: Atrial (Regular)* Irregular   Ventricular Regular (Irregular)

P WAVES: Upright PR: Variable QRS: 0.10s QT: 0.42s

ST SEGMENT: (Okay) Elevated Depressed   T WAVES: Upright

*Underlying rhythm

81.

Sinus rhythm with second degree type II AV block; Mobitz II; with downsloping ST depression

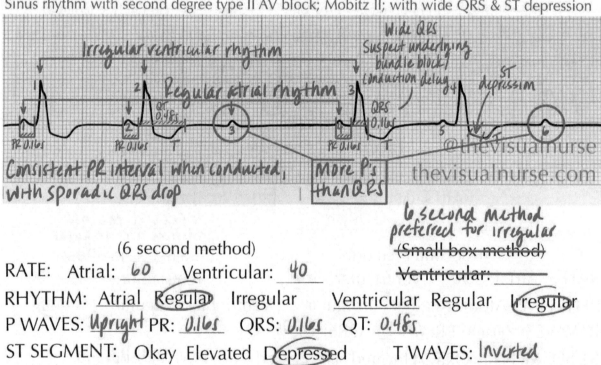

(6 second method)

RATE: Atrial: __80__ Ventricular: __50__   ~~Ventricular:~~ _____

RHYTHM: Atrial (Regular) Irregular   Ventricular Regular (Irregular)

P WAVES: Upright PR: __0.16s__ QRS: __0.08s__ QT: __0.32s__

ST SEGMENT: Okay Elevated (Depressed)   T WAVES: Inverted

82.

Sinus rhythm with second degree type II AV block; Mobitz II; with wide QRS & ST depression

(6 second method)

RATE: Atrial: __60__ Ventricular: __40__   ~~Ventricular:~~ _____

RHYTHM: Atrial (Regular) Irregular   Ventricular Regular (Irregular)

P WAVES: Upright PR: __0.16s__ QRS: __0.16s__ QT: __0.48s__

ST SEGMENT: Okay Elevated (Depressed)   T WAVES: Inverted

83.

Complete heart block; 3rd degree AV block

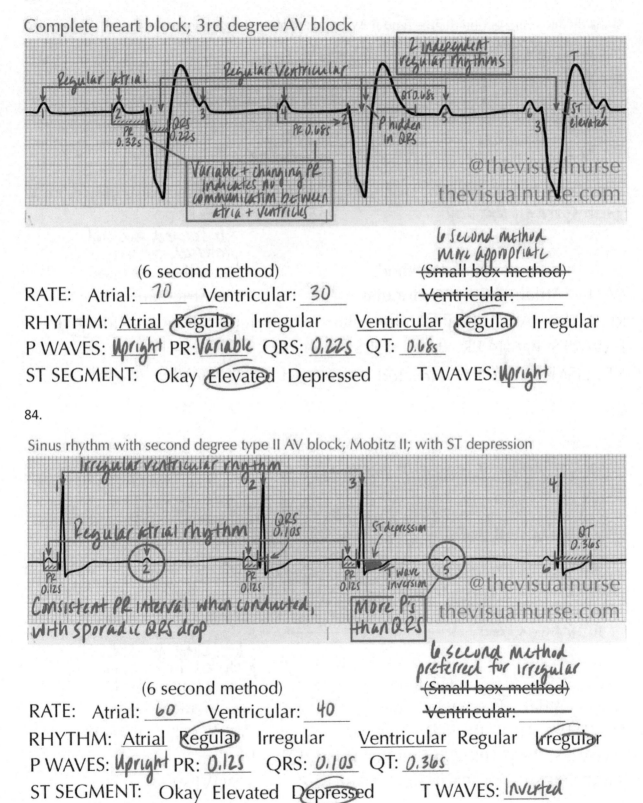

(6 second method)

6 second method more appropriate

(Small box method)

RATE: Atrial: 70   Ventricular: 30   Ventricular: _____

RHYTHM: Atrial (Regular) Irregular   Ventricular (Regular) Irregular

P WAVES: Upright PR: Variable QRS: 0.22s QT: 0.68s

ST SEGMENT: Okay (Elevated) Depressed   T WAVES: Upright

84.

Sinus rhythm with second degree type II AV block; Mobitz II; with ST depression

(6 second method)

6 second method preferred for irregular

(Small box method)

RATE: Atrial: 60   Ventricular: 40   Ventricular: _____

RHYTHM: Atrial (Regular) Irregular   Ventricular Regular (Irregular)

P WAVES: Upright PR: 0.12s   QRS: 0.10s   QT: 0.36s

ST SEGMENT: Okay Elevated (Depressed)   T WAVES: Inverted

85.

Sinus rhythm with second degree type II AV block; Mobitz II; with downsloping ST depression

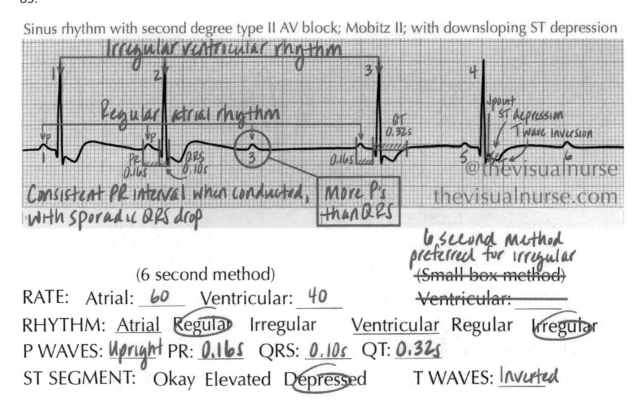

(6 second method)

RATE: Atrial: __60__   Ventricular: __40__   ~~Ventricular:~~ _____

RHYTHM: <u>Atrial</u> (Regular) Irregular   <u>Ventricular</u> Regular (Irregular)

P WAVES: <u>Upright</u> PR: **0.16s**   QRS: **0.10s**   QT: **0.32s**

ST SEGMENT: Okay Elevated (Depressed)   T WAVES: <u>Inverted</u>

86.

Sinus rhythm with a second degree type II AV block; Mobitz II

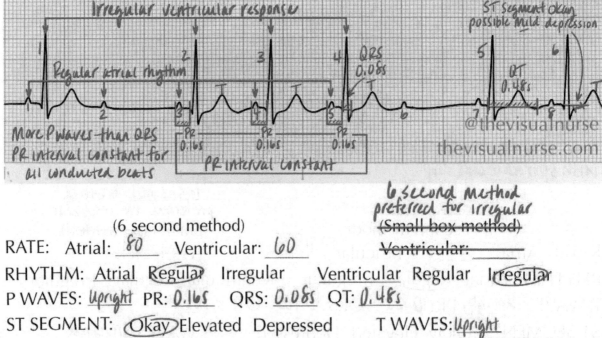

(6 second method)

RATE: Atrial: __80__   Ventricular: __60__   ~~Ventricular:~~ _____

RHYTHM: <u>Atrial</u> (Regular) Irregular   <u>Ventricular</u> Regular (Irregular)

P WAVES: <u>Upright</u> PR: **0.16s**   QRS: **0.08s**   QT: **0.48s**

ST SEGMENT: (Okay) Elevated Depressed   T WAVES: <u>Upright</u>

87.

Sinus rhythm with second degree type I AV block; Mobitz I; Wenckebach & downsloping ST depression

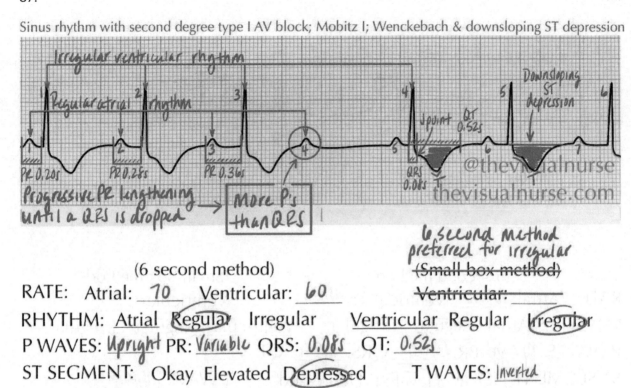

(6 second method)

RATE: Atrial: _70_ Ventricular: _60_   ~~Ventricular:~~ _____

RHYTHM: Atrial (Regular) Irregular   Ventricular Regular (Irregular)

P WAVES: Upright PR: Variable QRS: 0.08s QT: 0.52s

ST SEGMENT: Okay Elevated (Depressed)   T WAVES: Inverted

88.

Sinus rhythm with a wide QRS and second degree type II AV block; Mobitz II

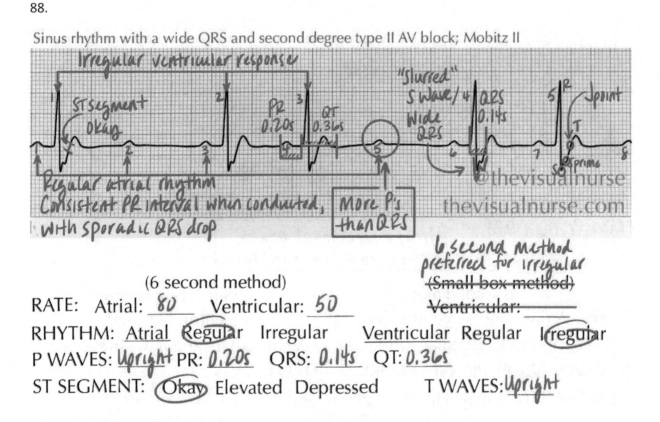

(6 second method)

RATE: Atrial: _80_ Ventricular: _50_   ~~Ventricular:~~ _____

RHYTHM: Atrial (Regular) Irregular   Ventricular Regular (Irregular)

P WAVES: Upright PR: 0.20s QRS: 0.14s QT: 0.36s

ST SEGMENT: (Okay) Elevated Depressed   T WAVES: Upright

89.

Complete heart block with ST elevation

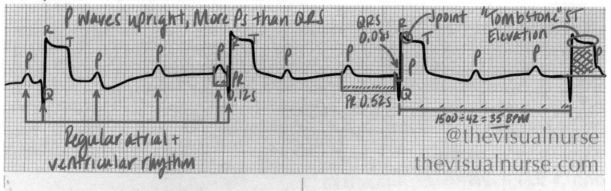

(6 second method)   (Small box method)

RATE: Atrial: _90-100_ Ventricular: _40_   Ventricular: _35_

RHYTHM: Atrial (Regular) Irregular   Ventricular (Regular) Irregular

P WAVES: Upright PR: Variable QRS: 0.08s QT: 0.32s

ST SEGMENT: Okay (Elevated) Depressed   T WAVES: Upright

90.

Complete heart block; 3rd degree AV block with downsloping ST depression

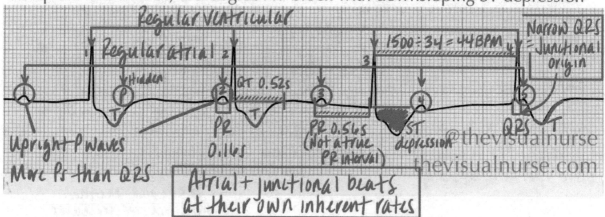

(6 second method)   (Small box method)

RATE: Atrial: _50_ Ventricular: _40_   Ventricular: _44_

RHYTHM: Atrial (Regular) Irregular   Ventricular (Regular) Irregular

P WAVES: Upright PR: Variable QRS: 0.06s QT: 0.52s

ST SEGMENT: Okay Elevated (Depressed)   T WAVES: Inverted

91.

Complete heart block; 3rd degree AV block with ST elevation

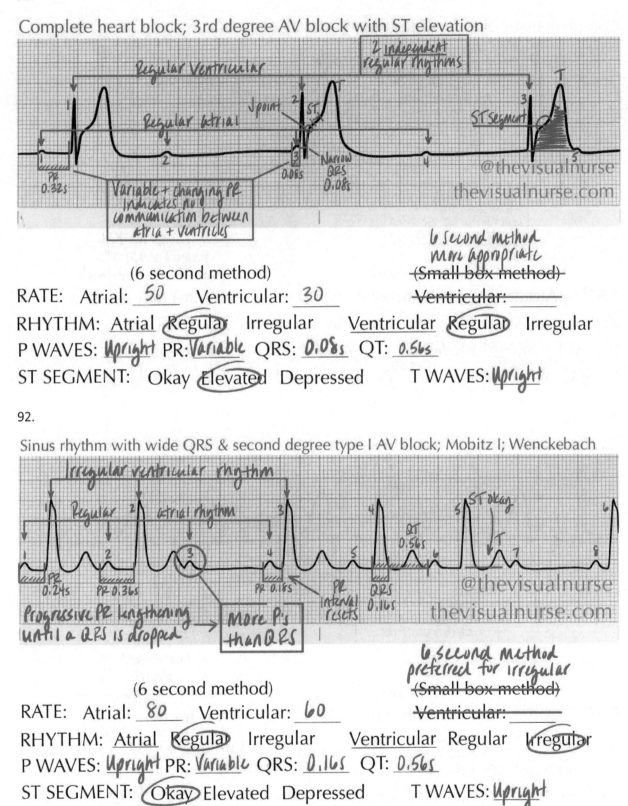

(6 second method)

RATE: Atrial: _50_ Ventricular: _30_   ~~(Small box method)~~ ~~Ventricular:~~____

RHYTHM: Atrial (Regular) Irregular   Ventricular (Regular) Irregular

P WAVES: Upright PR: Variable QRS: 0.08s QT: 0.56s

ST SEGMENT: Okay (Elevated) Depressed   T WAVES: Upright

92.

Sinus rhythm with wide QRS & second degree type I AV block; Mobitz I; Wenckebach

(6 second method)

RATE: Atrial: _80_ Ventricular: _60_   ~~(Small box method)~~ ~~Ventricular:~~____

RHYTHM: Atrial (Regular) Irregular   Ventricular Regular (Irregular)

P WAVES: Upright PR: Variable QRS: 0.16s QT: 0.56s

ST SEGMENT: (Okay) Elevated Depressed   T WAVES: Upright

93.

Complete heart block; 3rd degree AV block

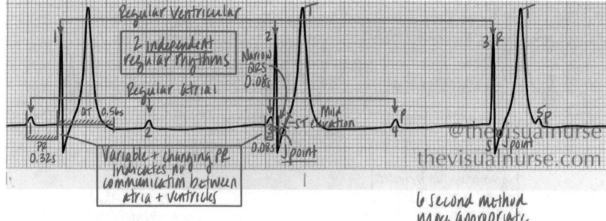

(6 second method)

RATE: Atrial: **50**   Ventricular: **30**   ~~(Small box method)~~ ~~Ventricular:~~ ____

6 second method more appropriate

RHYTHM: Atrial (Regular) Irregular   Ventricular (Regular) Irregular

P WAVES: **Upright** PR: **Variable** QRS: **0.08s** QT: **0.56s**

ST SEGMENT: Okay (Elevated) Depressed   T WAVES: **Upright**

94.

Complete heart block; 3rd degree AV block

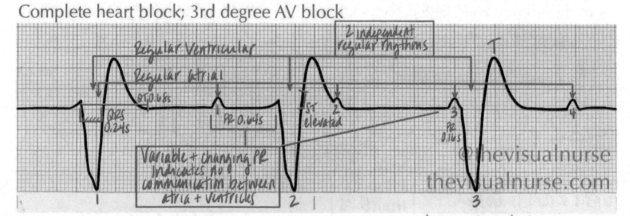

(6 second method)

RATE: Atrial: **40**   Ventricular: **30**   ~~(Small box method)~~ ~~Ventricular:~~ ____

6 second method more appropriate

RHYTHM: Atrial (Regular) Irregular   Ventricular (Regular) Irregular

P WAVES: **Upright** PR: **Variable** QRS: **0.24s** QT: **0.68s**

ST SEGMENT: Okay (Elevated) Depressed   T WAVES: **Upright**

95.

Atrial paced rhythm

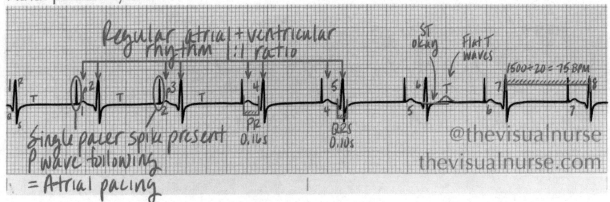

(6 second method)   (Small box method)
RATE: Atrial: _70_   Ventricular: _80_   Ventricular: _75_
RHYTHM: Atrial (Regular) Irregular   Ventricular (Regular) Irregular
P WAVES: Upright PR: _0.16s_ QRS: _0.10s_ QT: Unable to determine
ST SEGMENT: (Okay) Elevated Depressed   T WAVES: _Flat_

96.

Atrial paced rhythm

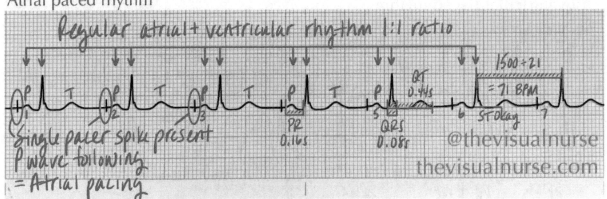

(6 second method)   (Small box method)
RATE: Atrial: _70_   Ventricular: _70_   Ventricular: _71_
RHYTHM: Atrial (Regular) Irregular   Ventricular (Regular) Irregular
P WAVES: Upright PR: _0.16s_ QRS: _0.08s_ QT: _0.44s_
ST SEGMENT: (Okay) Elevated Depressed   T WAVES: Upright

97.

Ventricular paced rhythm

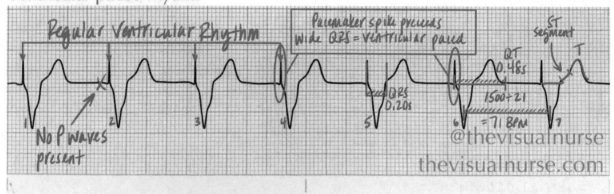

(6 second method) (Small box method)

RATE: Atrial: __NIA__ Ventricular: __70__ Ventricular: __71__

RHYTHM: ~~Atrial~~ ~~Regular~~ ~~Irregular~~ Ventricular (Regular) Irregular

P WAVES: __NIA__ PR: __NIA__ QRS: __0.20s__ QT: __0.48s__

ST SEGMENT: Okay (Elevated) Depressed T WAVES: __Upright__

98.

Atrioventricular paced rhythm

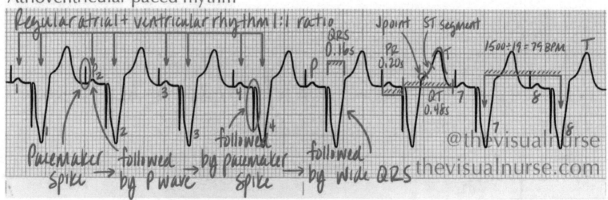

(6 second method) (Small box method)

RATE: Atrial: __80__ Ventricular: __80__ Ventricular: __79__

RHYTHM: Atrial (Regular) Irregular Ventricular Regular (Irregular)

P WAVES: __Upright__ PR: __0.20s__ QRS: __0.16s__ QT: __0.48s__

ST SEGMENT: Okay (Elevated) Depressed T WAVES: __Upright__

99.

Ventricular paced rhythm

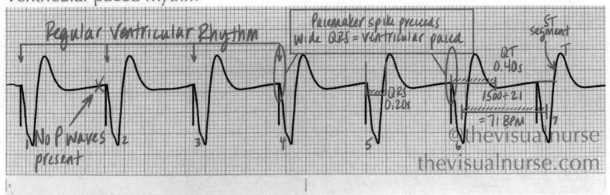

(6 second method)   (Small box method)

RATE: Atrial: _NIA_   Ventricular: _70_   Ventricular: _71_

RHYTHM: ~~Atrial~~ ~~Regular~~ ~~Irregular~~   Ventricular (Regular) Irregular

P WAVES: _NIA_ PR: _NIA_   QRS: _0.20s_ QT: _0.40s_

ST SEGMENT: Okay (Elevated) Depressed   T WAVES: _Upright_

100.

Atrioventricular paced rhythm

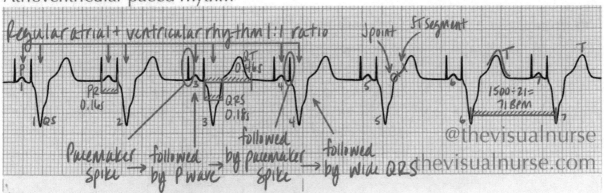

(6 second method)   (Small box method)

RATE: Atrial: _70_ Ventricular: _70_   Ventricular: _71_

RHYTHM: Atrial (Regular) Irregular   Ventricular (Regular) Irregular

P WAVES: _Upright_ PR: _0.16s_   QRS: _0.18s_ QT: _0.46s_

ST SEGMENT: Okay (Elevated) Depressed   T WAVES: _Upright_

101.

Atrial sensed, ventricular paced rhythm

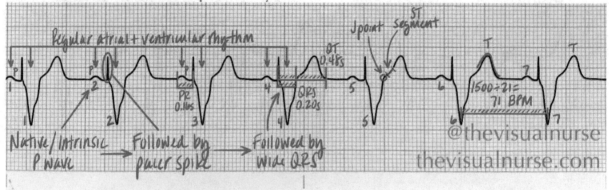

(6 second method)   (Small box method)
RATE: Atrial: _10_ Ventricular: _70_   Ventricular: _71_
RHYTHM: Atrial (Regular) Irregular   Ventricular (Regular) Irregular
P WAVES: Upright PR: 0.16s QRS: 0.20s QT: 0.48s
ST SEGMENT: Okay (Elevated) Depressed   T WAVES: Upright

102.

Ventricular paced rhythm with failure to capture

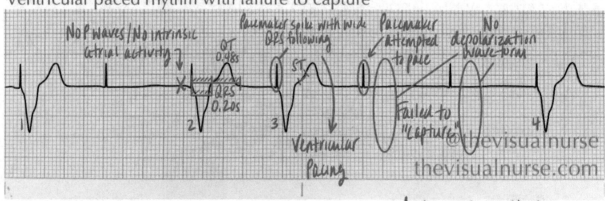

6 second method
preferred for irregular

(6 second method)   ~~(Small box method)~~
RATE: Atrial: _N/A_ Ventricular: _40_   ~~Ventricular:~~
RHYTHM: ~~Atrial Regular Irregular~~   Ventricular Regular (Irregular)
P WAVES: N/A PR: N/A QRS: 0.20s QT: 0.48s
ST SEGMENT: Okay (Elevated) Depressed   T WAVES: Upright

103.

Ventricular paced rhythm with failure to capture

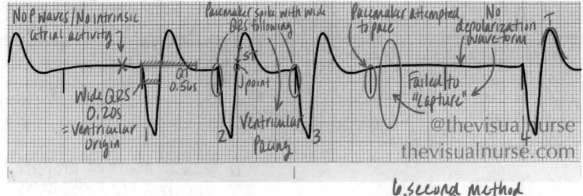

No P waves / No Intrinsic atrial activity
Wide QRS 0.20S = Ventricular Origin
Pacemaker spike with wide QRS following
ST
0.56s
J point
Ventricular Pacing
Pacemaker attempted to pace
No depolarization waveform
Failed to "capture"
@thevisualnurse
thevisualnurse.com

6 second method preferred for irregular
~~(Small box method)~~

(6 second method)

RATE: Atrial: N/A   Ventricular: 40   ~~Ventricular:~~

RHYTHM: ~~Atrial Regular Irregular~~ Ventricular Regular (Irregular)

P WAVES: N/A PR: N/A   QRS: 0.20S QT: 0.56s

ST SEGMENT: Okay (Elevated) Depressed   T WAVES: Upright

104.

Ventricular paced rhythm with failure to sense

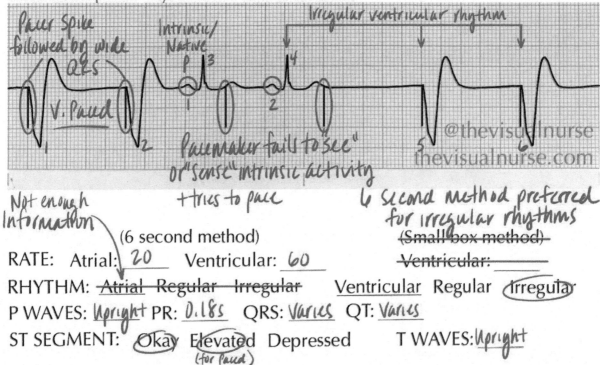

Pacer spike followed by wide QRS
V. Paced
Intrinsic/ Native P
Irregular ventricular rhythm
Pacemaker fails to "see" or "sense" intrinsic activity + tries to pace
@thevisualnurse
thevisualnurse.com

Not enough Information

6 second method preferred for irregular rhythms
~~(Small box method)~~

(6 second method)

RATE: Atrial: 20   Ventricular: 60   ~~Ventricular:~~

RHYTHM: ~~Atrial Regular Irregular~~ Ventricular Regular (Irregular)

P WAVES: Upright PR: 0.18s   QRS: Varies QT: Varies

ST SEGMENT: (Okay) Elevated Depressed   T WAVES: Upright
(for Paced)

105.

Ventricular paced with failure to pace

Irregular ventricular rhythm

Normal pacing resumes

Period of No pacemaker activity where pacer spikes should be

Pacemaker spike followed by wide QRS = V. Paced

Intrinsic ventricular beat occurs

@thevisualnurse
thevisualnurse.com

6 second method preferred for irregular rhythms

(6 second method)

(Small box method)

RATE: Atrial: N/A   Ventricular: 50   ~~Ventricular:~~

RHYTHM: ~~Atrial   Regular   Irregular~~   Ventricular Regular (Irregular)

P WAVES: N/A   PR: N/A   QRS: Wide/Variable   QT: Variable

ST SEGMENT: Okay (Elevated) Depressed   T WAVES: Upright

Made in the USA
Las Vegas, NV
19 December 2023

83244059R00077